ADVANCE PRAISE FOR *KRAV MAGA*

"Get in the best shape of your life while learning the most effective self-defense technique in the world."

—DAVID BARTON, RENOWNED FITNESS EXPERT AND OWNER, DAVID BARTON GYMS

"*Krav maga* is a name used to designate the Israel Defense Forces' original hand-to-hand combat system. *Krav maga*'s key training factor is to trim the time needed to condition a human being to prevail in a life-threatening situation where other armed people are the only obstacle to safety. David Kahn has spent many training hours in Israel and is also a good friend whom I met through the benevolent spirit of instructors of such skill."

—BOAZ AVIRAM, FORMER CHIEF KRAV MAGA INSTRUCTOR, ISRAEL DEFENSE FORCES FIGHTING FITNESS ACADEMY

"Training with *krav maga* instructor David Kahn was an honor and privilege. Having attended various self-defense and weapons retention courses, I was impressed with the power, grace, and economy of this training method. David's skills as a teacher and guide are second to none, and the tactics he teaches are a valuable skill that can help anyone detect, avoid, and if necessary prevail in a confrontation of any kind."

—MARK A. HANAFEE, U.S. COAST GUARD/POLICE TRAINING OFFICER

"*Krav maga* has been tested in real-life situations and gives you the knowledge to defuse a situation quickly. David Kahn is a wonderful teacher and I wholeheartedly recommend this book or his classes to anyone—male or female, big or small, or fat."

—JAMES GANDOLFINI, ACTOR (*THE SOPRANOS*)

KRAV MAGA

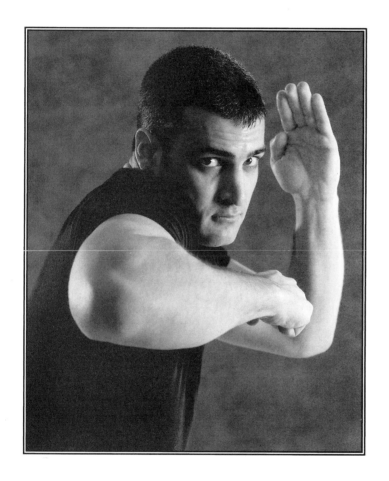

An Essential
Guide to the
Renowned
Method—
for Fitness and
Self-Defense

DAVID KAHN

ST. MARTIN'S GRIFFIN ✳ NEW YORK

This book is a tribute to the memory of krav maga
creator Emerich ("Imi") Lichtenfeld (1910–1998) and my own grandfathers of that great freedom-fighting generation. This book is further dedicated to all who uphold and safeguard our most cherished democratic values of freedom, equality, and tolerance.

www.stmartins.com

Design by Kathryn Parise
Illustrations by Precision Graphics

LIBRARY OF CONGRESS CATALOGING-IN-PUBLICATION DATA

Kahn, David, 1972–
    Krav maga : an essential guide to the renowned method—for fitness and self-defense / David Kahn.
      p. cm.
    ISBN 0-312-33177-0
    EAN 978-0312-33177-1
    1. Krav maga. 2. Self-defense. I. Title.

GV1111.K25 2004
796.8—dc22   2004046824

10 9 8 7

CONTENTS

ACKNOWLEDGMENTS

I am indebted to Grandmaster Haim Gidon for the training insights he provided as president of the Israeli Krav Maga Association (IKMA) and for the countless hours he spent with me on the mat. I am also indebted to my other Israeli *krav maga* instructors and good friends: Ohad, Albert, and Noam Gidon; Yoav Krayn; Yigal Arbiv; and Eran Buaron. Thanks to Michel Gidon for her hospitality and many meals spent at the grandmaster's table. Thanks to Aldema Zirinski for his indispensable support, advice and historical input. Thanks also to Maj. David Hassid of the Israeli Police Operational Fitness Academy. I am grateful to the IKMA (Israeli Krav Maga Association) Board of Directors and all IKMA members who have welcomed and trained with me over the years. This book would not be possible without the expert training, support, and inspiration provided by the Israeli Krav Maga Association.

To senior *krav maga* instructor and technical language advisor, Rick Blitstein, I am forever grateful for our chance meeting under the *sukkah* that set this book in motion. I am grateful to historical contributor Boaz Aviram, former Israel Defense Forces (IDF) *krav maga* chief military instructor, for his support and insights. I am grateful to security instructor and counterterror expert Nir Maman for his support and contributions. To my Philadelphia training partners, Alan Feldman, Ken Winokur, Neil Greenberg, Allen Opalek, and Al Ackerman, thank you for helping to send me on my way. Thanks to the South American Krav Maga Association and Manchester Maccabi Krav Maga for their support. Thanks to my uncle David Kahn for carrying on the *krav maga* instructor tradition. I am thankful to Capt. Peter Savalli, Chief Anthony Gaylord, Trooper Paul Miller, Mark Hanafee, Kevin Colon, Eric Givens, and all of the other dedicated men and women of American law enforcement who protect us and have welcomed *krav maga* training.

Special thanks goes to David Barton for his unparalleled support, along with his staff, and for introducing me to my special training partner, Bailey Barton. I am equally appreciative of the 92nd St. Y Makor organization's efforts in helping to build *krav maga*. To IKMA instructors, Rich Felsher, Sean Quimby, Brian Linnet, Dr. Peter Rosenthal, Elizabeth Greenman, and Ethan Vogelhut, thank you for your invaluable support in expanding *krav maga*. Thanks to WR Mann of www.RealFighting.com for his indispensable guidance and support. Many thanks go to my good friends and training partners, Bill and Justin Kingson, for their insights and effort. Thanks to Dr. Steven R. Gecha for keeping me in one piece over the many years. Thanks to my best friend, Brian E. Goldberg, for his support and legal counsel. Thanks to Dr. Ari Malka for his support and insight. To my sharp-elbowed Makor women, Shari, Ariela, and Katherina, thanks for their dedication and for beating me up to show it works. Thanks to Greg Holland for his support and interest. Thanks to Emmy and Golden Globe Award–winning actor James Gandolfini for his public support.

Special thanks go to my family for their unwaivering support of my *krav maga* training and the hospitality extended to my Israeli instructors. Much thanks goes to my mother, Anne, for her comma checking and to my grandmother, Helen, for feeding us all and sending me packing each time with sustenance to Netanya. I am grateful to my father, Alfred, for encouraging my many trips to Israel and for my brother Abel playing the role of "assailant" so many times to help us build *krav maga*. I thank my uncle Harry for toughening me up and my stepfather, Ed, for being the voice of reason in this undertaking. Vanessa, thank you for your devotion and contributions.

Last, I would like to thank the wonderful group of St. Martin's Press and Alisa Bauman for making this book come alive. A heartfelt thanks goes to my editor, Marian Lizzi, for recognizing the need for a book on the fundamentals of Israeli self-defense.

INTRODUCTION

Why I Love *Krav Maga*— and Why You Will, Too

Discover how Israeli self-defense
can save your life

My introduction to Israeli *krav maga* floored me—literally. Soon after beginning law school, I met Israeli Krav Maga Association (IKMA) senior instructor Rick Blitstein. Rick sat reading quietly at a table. I noticed his T-shirt first. On it in big, bold letters were the words, ISRAELI *KRAV MAGA* MARTIAL ARTS. I was curious.

I asked, "What does 'Israeli *krav maga*' mean?"

Rick sized me up and said, "*Krav maga* is the official fighting system of the Israeli military." He went on to explain the merits and benefits of *krav maga* telling me that it is a system unlike any other. From that moment, I was hooked.

Until that time I had managed to stay fit by playing football. At the end of my football career, however, I needed another fitness hobby to pursue. I wanted to explore a self-defense program that would not only teach hard-core self-defense, but also keep me in shape. I also wanted a program that I could notch up or down as I saw fit. I remembered that initial conversation with Rick and decided to explore what *krav maga* had to offer. I'm very glad I did. *Krav maga* has given me all of that—and much more.

During my first class, Rick decided to use me as a would-be assailant. As I stood waiting to see what would happen, I don't remember feeling particularly vulnerable. Even after my football career, I was still lifting weights. I stood 6 feet tall and weighed about 200 pounds. I looked down on Rick, who was about an inch or two shorter and about forty pounds lighter. If you saw both of us on the street and knew nothing of our background, you probably would have bet that I could easily take him in a confrontation.

Rick asked me to come at him. The next thing I remember, I was lying on the floor and Rick was standing over me. "What just happened?" I wondered as I looked up at him in a daze. He grinned down at me. Eventually I got to my feet, moved to the back of the practice line, and silently marveled at the simplicity of Rick's technique. The genius behind the *krav maga* system dawned on me in that moment. I wanted what Rick had—and I subsequently have spent the next ten years building my *krav maga* skills, techniques, and fitness. Now I want to introduce you to this efficient, effective, and empowering system.

What *Krav Maga* Can Do for You

Krav maga has provided me with confidence and peace of mind. I am confident when I must walk down a dark, deserted street or when confronted by menacing strangers. If necessary, I am trained to defend myself against any attacker of any size or skill level. I want you to gain some of that same confidence.

You may be your own first and last line of defense in an increasingly violent world. The best law-enforcement and security agencies in the world cannot be everywhere at all times. The attacks of September 11, 2001, and terrorism's global scourge confirm the vulnerability we all face as ordinary citizens. Whether the threat comes from a mugger, rapist, or terrorist, your life is at

FIGHTING FIT ↙

Dr. Ari Malka was an overweight child, weighing approximately 250 pounds at his high school graduation. Over the years since high school, he tried to lose weight many times, but the weight didn't budge. That is, until he discovered *krav maga*. Ari is now a 170-pound lean, mean fighting machine who has trained with me, as well as with Rick Blitstein and Grandmaster Haim Gidon in Israel.

"I finally found what I was looking for," Ari says. "*Krav maga* is a self-defense and fitness discipline made for everyone. As a physician, I cannot imagine a form of physical activity better suited to the general public." Ari says he walks away from every class with a sense of accomplishment, satisfaction, and self-improvement. Even when he cannot physically train, he practices *krav maga* by spending a few minutes stretching, shadow boxing, and running through techniques in his head.

"I walk with a heightened sense of alertness wherever I am, and I feel confident handling all types of potential confrontation," he says. "I learned skills in avoiding potential danger and diffusing situations early. If all else fails, I know I can count on my knowledge of self-defense. *Krav maga* has helped me so much throughout the last several years, keeping me grounded, physically fit, confident, and happy. I recommend the system to all those interested in personal security as well as those, who like me, are simply looking for a fun way to get in shape."

↙

stake. You must be prepared to do whatever it takes to survive. There are no rules on the street.

Battle-tested and street-proven, Israeli *krav maga,* which translates to "contact combat," is the Israel Defense Force's official self-defense and close-quarters-combat system. Based on utility, instinct, simplicity, and adaptability, the Israeli *krav maga* system is one of the most effective, practical, and holistic fighting systems in the world. *Krav maga* will condition your body, mind, and soul.

Krav maga benefits people of all shapes, sizes, and physical abilities regardless of age. For example, learning to fall backward without smashing your head or breaking your tailbone is important for everyone, including the elderly and children. Although *krav maga* was designed to teach soldiers to become proficient in close-quarters-combat tactics in a short time, its techniques apply to civilians as well. In addition, it is now becoming increasingly popular as a conditioning and fitness regimen, and you will see why.

Throughout the pages of this book, you will learn more than one hundred techniques designed to keep you safe in the most common unarmed street encounters. From punches to kicks, eye gouges to groin strikes, you'll not only learn how to defend yourself and keep your attacker away, but you'll also learn how to control, subdue, and maim your attacker if necessary. In Chapter 9 of this book, you'll embark on a twelve-week training plan designed to transform even the smallest, frailest, weakest, and least confident person into a fit, confident, and fight-ready *kravist.*

By the end of your twelve-week plan, you will . . .

- be able to instinctively defend against strikes from a myriad of angles;
- be able to release from grabs, hair pulls, and chokes from all angles;
- be consciously aware of your surroundings, safety, and impending danger, recognizing danger sooner so that you will be able to anticipate and ideally prevent an attack from happening;

- have increased hand/eye and right-side/left-side body co-
ordinations;
- and be in the best shape of your life.

Yes, that's right, *krav maga* training will improve your overall
fitness. But to learn *krav maga* and gain its fitness benefits, plus be
able to employ it instinctively, you must practice. Your practice
will include a rigorous workout using continuous-motion self-
defense, close-quarters-combat techniques. You'll strengthen
every major muscle group in your body. As you practice punching
and other upper body techniques, you will strengthen your arms,
chest, upper back, and shoulders. Similarly, your kicks and lower
body techniques will strengthen your legs, hips, and buttocks. In

The Core Curriculum

Many gyms are pushing a popular concept and training regimen
known as "core fitness" these days. For these exercise programs,
you emphasize the core muscles of the body in the abdomen, hips,
and back. In addition to helping you to flatten your tummy and
sculpt a 6-pack, this core focus also helps you build strength in
your power centers: the abdomen and hips. When you move from
your abdomen and hips, you gain more power for all of your fitness
pursuits, from running to tennis to *krav maga*.

   Krav maga builds core strength. The stronger your core muscles, the better able you'll be able to put all of your body weight
behind your punches, kicks, and other strikes. Conversely, the more
you put your entire body behind your strikes, the stronger your core
will become. *Krav maga* builds core strength in many other ways as
well. Kicking requires balance and coordination as you lift and
extend your leg. Each time you kick, you build core strength as muscles throughout your abdomen work to keep you upright.

krav maga every movement requires you to use your core—your abdomen and back—as you place the weight of your entire body behind every strike. You will practice punching, kicking, and other techniques against pads to build strength, shadow boxing to build your cardiovascular capacity, and partner sparring to fine tune your reaction time, balance, cardiovascular fitness, and core strength. *Krav maga* training will keep you lean, agile, and fit. Staying lean, agile, and fit will help you to become a better *krav-ist.* Although you can successfully employ certain techniques with only a minimum amount of fitness, your *krav maga* training can certainly soon become your primary fitness pursuit. Although I still run and lift weights, *krav maga* has become my primary workout. I need only practice my techniques fifteen to twenty minutes a day to stay in top shape—and keep my skills sharp at the same time.

My *Krav Maga* Background

I've devoted much of my adult life to the study—and eventual teaching—of *krav maga.* After three years of nonstop *krav maga* training with Rick Blitstein during law school, I wanted to experience the system in its highest form. To do so, I traveled to *krav maga*'s source: the Israeli Krav Maga Association (IKMA), located in creator Imi Lichtenfeld's hometown, Netanya, Israel. I had the privilege of arriving at Grandmaster Haim Gidon's doorstep to begin a customized instructor certification course, the first of many special training visits. I was not sure what to expect, but the level of expertise exhibited in the grandmaster's gym was simply awe inspiring. The grandmaster's movements were just unbelievable. Haim anticipated his opponent's movements before they happened. His senior instructors were no less formidable. Even beginner students looked as if they could take on the world.

I eventually earned my black-belt advanced teaching certifications from Grandmaster Haim Gidon and now sit on the Israeli Krav Maga Association's Board of Directors. I now teach *krav maga* at the David Barton Gyms and the 92nd St. Y Makor organization. We also instruct federal, state, and local law-enforcement agencies in the method. Through the Israeli Krav Maga Association, I now receive requests from all over the world to teach *krav maga*. Along with others in the association, I have taught *krav maga* to people of all shapes and sizes, ages, and backgrounds, including celebrities, CEOs, fitness buffs, the elderly, children, and victims of violent crimes. They all appreciate the confidence that *krav maga* training develops. Time and time again, students tell us how amazed they feel about their mind and body transformation. In teaching them *krav maga*, we have not only taught them how to successfully defend themselves, we've also taught them how to build better coordination, balance, and hand-eye coordination. For example, we build games into the children's curriculum to keep them energetic, teach them discipline, and instill a sense of respect for adults and their peers. For the elderly, we've developed a modified training program that helps them stay fit and active. My passion is to both learn and teach *krav maga*. I hope to share this passion with you.

Krav maga has impacted my life and the lives of thousands of other practitioners in countless ways, enhancing body, mind, and soul. I've been extremely lucky during my life and have not had to use my *krav maga* skills often. Many of my family members and students, on the other hand, have called upon their *krav maga* skills during various confrontations. You'll read their inspiring stories throughout the pages of this book.

Confidence in the *krav maga* system builds confidence in yourself. Perhaps the most beneficial skill I have learned from *krav maga* is how to extricate myself from a threatening situation without force. For example, once while traveling by subway, a man sitting near me mistakenly thought I had said something vulgar to his wife. He yelled at me, "I am going to slit your throat." I assumed a defensive stance and calmly but forcefully said, "I now consider you a threat to my life and am prepared to act accordingly. You are in my danger zone." He and his wife quickly walked away without an incident.

My *krav maga* training has benefited me in many other important ways. For example, a few years ago, a car hit me as I was riding my bike. Thanks to my *krav maga* training, I reacted quickly and instinctively. I jumped off the bike as the car made impact, preventing my knees from getting crushed. I rolled onto the hood of the car and across the windshield. Later, medics at the scene marveled that I was still alive and mostly unharmed by the accident. Had I not been trained in *krav maga*, I would have reacted differently, resulting in potentially serious injury.

Learning *krav maga* might prevent the unacceptable from happening to you and your loved ones. Hopefully, you will never need these skills, and in the words of *krav maga* founder Imi Lichtenfeld, you may always "walk in peace." Nevertheless, you will be prepared should the need for self-defense arise. Anyone can learn *krav maga*. Everyone *should* learn *krav maga*.

Frequently Asked Questions

Over the years I've been asked many questions from potential students about *krav maga*. Perhaps some of these same questions are swimming through your mind right now. Below you'll find my answers to the most frequently asked questions about *krav maga*.

Q: *To train in* krav maga, *do I need previous self-defense training?*

A: No. *Krav maga* is designed for everyone to learn self-defense and fighting skills regardless of previous self-defense training. *Krav maga*'s overriding philosophy is to do "whatever works." While *krav maga* emphasizes several basic techniques and advanced technique variations to neutralize a dangerous situation, there is no absolute or correct answer. The system is flexible, true to its modern combat evolution. Techniques are constantly modified, revised, added, and discarded as real-life encounters are taken into account and analyzed.

Q: *Will I need a uniform or specific training attire?*

A: No. *Krav maga* does not require traditional martial arts attire or uniforms. For practical purposes, however, practitioners are encouraged to wear athletic attire. Many *krav maga* practitioners like to wear a *krav maga* shirt for class spirit and uniformity. In Israel, IKMA or solid-colored shirts are usually worn along with white or black gee training pants. Athletic shoes, preferably flat-soled tennis or cross-trainer-type sneakers, or martial arts shoes are recommended. When specialized mats are used, the appropriate type of footwear is required. Male participants should wear protective athletic supporters, and some students choose to use mouth guards.

Q: *How are* krav maga *classes run?*

A: In the United States *krav maga* classes generally run from one hour to one and a half hours. Advanced seminars run longer. In Israel, the typical IKMA student trains six to eight hours per week.

I personally teach according to the Israeli curriculum. Classes begin with warm-ups and stretching, which prepares the body for the combative movements that follow. We practice the techniques in continuous motion with one technique blending into the next. Called *retzev,* this type of continuous-motion training simulates real-life encounters.

Grandmaster Haim Gidon and senior instructors will demonstrate techniques for the appropriate belt levels at full speed and will then break down and isolate each technique into its component parts. Students will then engage in the techniques. If a particular question catches the instructor's attention as something that will benefit the entire class, drills will temporarily halt for the instructor to provide further clarification and explanation. Classes in the United States follow the same basic format.

Q: *Do classes incorporate full-contact fighting?*

A: Yes and no. *Krav maga*, because of its nature, must be practiced under controlled conditions. Because striking at the body's vulnerable parts is *krav maga*'s underlying counterattack principle, you must use caution when applying techniques that target the groin, throat, eyes, and other vulnerable areas. Controlled sparring with varying degrees of power, while using protective gear, clinches, throws, and groundwork, are an integral part of the curriculum. Advanced students regularly participate in "fighting classes," using *krav maga* techniques to spar and grapple and do other partner work.

Q: *Are there any rules when practicing* krav maga?

A: Yes and no. *Krav maga* instructors emphasize two paradoxical but necessary training rules: (1) there are no rules in a fight, but (2) one must not injure oneself or one's partner when training.

Q: *Does* krav maga *distinguish training between men and women?*

A: No. Imi designed *krav maga* for people of all shapes, sizes, and physical abilities, regardless of age or gender. The same *krav maga* techniques, with minor modifications, are taught to men and women alike; however, the emphasis placed on certain techniques can be different. Size, strength, and reach are factors a defender—male or female—must take into consideration. This is especially true where one's limb reach is a determining factor. Often women are confronted with a predatory attack, which brings the attacker close. As a result, "infighting," using elbows, knees, eye gouges, and, if necessary, bites is emphasized. In addition, some women (and men) are reluctant to use their knuckles and hands for striking and, instead, may feel more comfortable, for example, using a palm heel. Several specially adapted *krav maga* ground-fighting techniques also address sexual predation and other dangers women may specifically face. You'll learn many of these techniques in this book.

Q: *Is* krav maga *training appropriate for children and adolescents?*

A: Yes. *Krav maga* is recognized by the Israeli Ministry of Education as the leading method of self-defense. The IKMA runs extensive training programs for children. Basic *krav maga* movements are taught, combining physical fitness training along with civic virtues. For example, we incorporate games into children's classes to build a sense of discipline and respect.

Q: *Does* krav maga *incorporate weapons defenses?*

A: Yes. *Krav maga* is world renowned for its weapons defenses, including threats from edged weapons, blunt weapons, firearms, and even microexplosives. In this book, however, we will focus on the fundamental techniques and principles of unarmed attack.

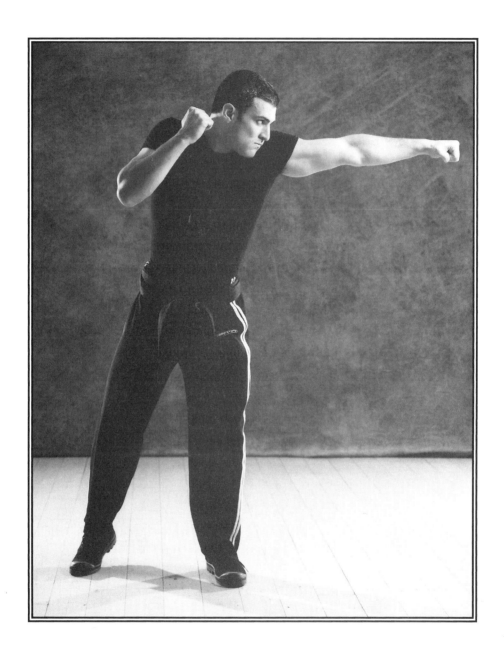

CHAPTER 1

The Power of Israeli *Krav Maga*

Gain confidence, personal safety, and overall fitness with the Israeli military's time-tested, self-defense system

When my brother Abel was twenty-eight, he set off for a solo backpacking trip around the world. He knew his two years of *krav maga* training would provide both physical security and a mental state of ease. He did not anticipate, however, how often he would find himself facing aggressors.

One day, while touring an open-air war museum in Hue, Vietnam, Abel walked past a large group of schoolboys huddled over gambling cards between two inoperable American tanks. As Abel passed the group, some of the boys jumped up and aggressively encircled him. Abel sensed a boy behind him, eyeing his pockets. As he felt the boy's index finger jab for his wallet, Abel quickly grabbed the child's finger, and, with an upward twisting motion against the child's finger joint, Abel spun to face him. He assumed physical control over the youth without hurting him, and the other youths scattered.

Later during that same trip, Abel was walking toward a beach when a young, muscular man charged toward him. The man flailed his arms and shouted aggressively. Abel knew the aggressor would close the gap between them within two to three seconds. Instinctively summoning his *krav maga* training, Abel pivoted on his feet, shifted his body weight, and prepared to kick his assailant. Fortunately, the man quickly turned in the other direction and walked away as he muttered, "Crazy American."

Krav maga, the Israel Defense Forces's official self-defense and close-quarters-combat system, can provide you with the same confidence and safety it has provided me, my brother, and the scores of students I have trained in the method. You need not be tall, strong, or burly to master the system. Indeed, Abel has successfully used *krav maga* in many situations. Many of my smallest, slightest, and even most elderly students have mastered *krav maga* and used it to escape dangerous situations. You'll read some of their inspiring stories throughout this book.

You also need not spend years mastering the techniques. With consistent training of about three to four hours a week, you can master some of *krav maga*'s most effective mental and physical techniques within roughly twelve weeks. You can perfect individual techniques much faster, in as little as 5 minutes as I have taught some of my students to successfully defend themselves. In addition to learning how to defend yourself in any situation at any time, you'll improve your fitness. You'll learn how to practice the *krav maga* techniques as a sequenced, heart-pumping routine. This not only will train your body to summon the energy when under pressure but also will . . .

- → condition your heart and lungs, reducing your risk for heart disease,

- improve your overall strength and muscle tone,
- allow you to generate explosive power,
- and help you to lose weight.

Simply stated, it's one of the most effective workouts around.

The Birth of *Krav Maga*

Krav maga is based on our most primitive and natural instincts. The Hebrew word *krav* means "struggle" and was first used in the Old Testament in the second book of Samuel, 17:11. *Maga* means "close" or "contact." Although many *krav maga* building-block techniques have existed for thousands of years, the self-defense system was developed, modernized, and fine-tuned during World War II and Israel's War of Independence by Emerich "Imi" Lichtenfeld (Imi Sde-Or).

Born in 1910 in Budapest, Hungary, Imi grew up in Bratislava, Czechoslovakia. Imi's father, Samuel Lichtenfeld, joined a professional circus troupe, where he excelled in both wrestling and boxing. After developing extensive knowledge in fitness training along with wrestling, boxing, and mixed-skill fighting, Samuel joined the Czech police as a detective and led the force in arrests.

Samuel founded and ran the wrestling club and gym Hercules, where he trained Imi and other young competitive athletes. Imi rapidly distinguished himself as a champion in judo, boxing, wrestling, gymnastics, and ballroom dancing, among other athletic pursuits. Imi also became a world-class gymnast, trained a ballet-dancing troupe, and starred as a stage show thespian in *Mephisto*.

In 1935 Imi visited Palestine with a team of Jewish wrestlers to compete in the Jewish Maccabi sports convention. Unfortunately, Imi fractured a rib during a training accident and could not compete. This accident led to Imi's fundamental training principle emphasized in his own words: "Don't get hurt." Imi quickly concluded that only real necessity justifies a "win at all costs" approach. These two tenets eventually fused to create Imi's *krav maga* training approach.

Imi returned to Czechoslovakia to face increasing anti-Semitic violence. As Nazi hatred infected Slovakia, Jews were increasingly victims of near-constant violence. To protect the Jewish community from marauding Fascists and anti-Semites, Imi organized a group of young Jews to protect his community. On the streets Imi quickly learned the vital differences between sport martial arts competition and street fighting. While serving on the front lines to protect his community, Imi began to combine natural movements and reactions with immediate and decisive counterattacks.

These community self-defense activities made Imi a wanted man by the Fascist Nazi occupational authorities. Nazi intolerance soon quickly reached a crescendo as the Germans began their systematic extermination of European Jewry. In May 1940 the Beitar Zionist Youth movement invited Imi to join them on the riverboat, *Pentcho,* bound for Palestine.

Imi steamed down the Danube through the hostile yet unoccupied banks of Hungary, Croatia, Yugoslavia, Bulgaria, and Romania and then into the open Black Sea through the Turkish Straits. He and other refugees survived the hardships of man and nature, including a quarantine intended to starve them while marooned on the Romanian delta. Imi showed his selflessness by plunging into the water and saving a drowning child. Consequently he developed an ear infection that would plague him throughout his journey.

Upon entering the Aegean Sea, the *Pentcho*'s engines failed, grounding the boat on a desolate island. Imi and three other refugees took a lifeboat and rowed for three days. Imi's ear infection gradually worsened and became life threatening. A British airplane spotted them and summoned a British warship to rescue them. After receiving treatment for his ear infection, Imi enlisted in the British-supervised Free Czech Legion. After exemplary military service in the Middle East, Imi was released from the British army following the German Afrika Korp's defeat at El Alamein in 1942. Imi was granted permission to remain in British-ruled Palestine. His friends then introduced him to the leaders of the Zionist community's defense organizations. Although Imi escaped to Palestine, his family remained behind. They all died during the war.

Israel's early leaders recognized Imi's fighting abilities, innovativeness, and his ability to impart this training to others. Imi began training the *Palmach* (elite strike force), the *Palyam* (marine commandos), and the *Haganah,* which would merge into the modern-day *Zahal* or Israel Defense Forces. This training included fighting fitness, obstacle training, bayonet tactics, sentry removal, knife fighting, stave/stick fighting, and any other military-oriented problems that required a creative solution.

In 1948 Imi became the principal authority on close-quarters combat for the Israel Defense Forces (IDF). He was in charge of training a disparate group of soldiers of all shapes, sizes, and abilities, many of whom did not speak the same language. He needed to develop a self-defense system that would work for not only spry eighteen year olds and elite fighting troops in prime physical condition but also for middle-aged and graying reserve soldiers. He needed a system that soldiers could learn quickly, during their three-week-long basic training. Finally, he needed a system that worked, one that soldiers could apply to any situation at any time intuitively and without hesitation.

A Fighting System That Works for All

Until the World War II era, traditional self-defense techniques often left soldiers ill-prepared to defend against armed attackers. As the fledging Israeli state formed, Imi knew its soldiers needed to learn a type of close-quarters combat that could protect them against firearms, explosives, and other modern threats. Thus, *krav maga*—the world's most effective close-quarters-combat system—was born.

As he developed the method, Imi worked tirelessly to ensure that *krav maga*'s success was not dependent on a practitioner's strength or expertise in any one combative. A combative consists of any manner of strikes, take downs, joint locks, chokes, ground fighting, or combined evasive action. He took all aspects of a fight, both armed and unarmed, into account.

Merging Self-Defense with Close-Quarters Combat

Until the advent of *krav maga,* self-defense and close-quarters combat were often thought of as two distinct methodologies. Self-defense usually included situations in which a defender was unaware of an impending attack. In close-quarters combat, two opponents are aware of the other's respective movements and perceived violent intent. *Krav maga* fuses the two disciplines into one fighting system, giving you the tools needed to defend yourself both when taken by surprise or when you are aware of your opponent. In *krav maga,* you'll learn to quickly react under *any* situation. You'll learn to both neutralize an attacker as well as develop a fight strategy that may include defensive posturing and movements, coordinated attacks and counterattacks, and overall tactics.

Imi had studied many different fighting styles in his youth, including boxing, wrestling, judo, jujitsu, aikido, and fencing. In 1948 Imi melded his knowledge of these various fighting disciplines together and created the complete fighting system now known as *krav maga*. The fledgling Israel Defense Forces (IDF) immediately recognized his system and formally adopted it because of its . . .

Simplicity *Krav maga* techniques are easy to learn and execute. Imi knew the Israel Defense Forces (IDF) needed a simple, fluid system, one that could readily incorporate modification and change and be mastered quickly, usually within three weeks of basic training. Similarly, if you follow the intensive training schedule outlined in subsequent chapters, you, too, can learn the system's basics in a short period of time.

Instinctive Nature To successfully fend off an attacker, you must move instinctively. Any delay or split-second hesitation can result in deadly consequences. Indeed, this is why *krav maga* relics on your natural instincts and rcflcxcs. *Krav maga* trains both your body and mind to effectively react to any threat without hesitation. Not only do you learn physical skills, such as punches and kicks, you also learn how to train your mind and overall defensive awareness. By recognizing situations and body language, you will perceive danger earlier and react to it sooner. In most cases, your *krav maga* training will help you to escape dangerous situations without ever having to employ your physical skills.

Utility An attack can come from a myriad angles and combinations. Imi created just a few defensive techniques that any trainee could master and apply to defend a spectrum of attacks. *Krav maga* will teach you to focus on a series of attack points, targeting your opponent's vulnerable vital points and applying your physical skills in an intuitive manner. You'll learn a core set of offensive techniques that will help you to overcome any number of an opponent's anticipated defenses. It's as if you are engaged in a fighting chess game. Optimally you'll sense and overcome your opponent's move before he can make it.

Use of Weapons of Opportunity   The *krav maga* techniques easily incorporate the use of firearms, knives, and various weapons of opportunity, such as loose change, keys, pens, cell phones, a belt buckle, or, even, spittle. You will learn how to use these everyday items to defend yourself in Chapter 4. That said, you will learn close-quarters combat as well and how to successfully defend yourself in unarmed situations.

Adaptability   Although you will learn tried and true mental and physical techniques and practice them regularly, your personal *krav maga* will become whatever most efficiently delivers you from harm's way. Imi astutely grasped the crucial difference between sport and street combat: rules or the lack of them. Sports contests are exactly that because rules create the game. Traditional martial arts competitions similarly require rules for contest and safety purposes. Fighting for your life is no game. To stay safe, you must give up any notion of fair play. Dislodging an attacker's eyeball or delivering a swift kick to the groin are viable and emphasized *krav maga* options, when the level of threat requires it.

Proficiency   *Krav maga* techniques are efficient, decisive, and effective.

During the 1950s and 1960s, Imi served as chief physical fitness and *krav maga* instructor for the Israel Defense Forces. The vast knowledge acquired through *krav maga* training prompted the military authorities to recognize *krav maga* as a distinct self-defense, close-quarters-combat system. Later the Israeli Ministry of Education also granted *krav maga* state recognition for training in public schools.

From Soldiers to Civilians

Imi's teaching skills were often sought abroad. His lessons extended beyond just self-defense, and close-quarters combat training to emphasize character and moral training. For example, in 1960, when instructing a Royal Police Guard unit in Ethiopia, Imi

---

About Grandmaster Haim Gidon

Grandmaster Haim Gidon (tenth *dan* and IKMA president) was born in Istanbul, Turkey, in 1944 and moved to Israel in 1961. Haim fought in the Six Day War, the War of Attrition, and the Yom Kippur War. Prior to the 1967 war, Haim resumed his competitive boxing and decided to learn more about the *krav maga* principles he had learned in the military. In 1978 Haim helped Imi cofound the IKMA.

In 1994 Haim was elected as IKMA president and opened his current gym and the main training center for the IKMA, located on Ben Zion Street, Netanya, Israel. In 1995 Imi entrusted Haim to grant 1st *dan* (black-belt levels) *krav maga* and senior dan levels. In a 1996 IKMA public ceremony, Imi awarded Haim Gidon 8th *dan,* and promised that 9th and 10th *dans* "were to come" and designating him as Imi's successor.

Imi approved of Haim's additions and modifications to the *krav maga* system, especially the development of *retzev* (fluid continuous movement), the extensive groundwork and weapons defense modifications.

Haim is a member of Israel's national Wingate Sports Institute's Professional Committee. He has taught *krav maga* tactics for the last thirty years to Israel's law-enforcement, security, and military personnel. He has received special commendation from federal, state, and local law-enforcement agencies worldwide for his specific *krav maga* professional law training curriculum. His teaching expertise is requested worldwide.

realized during a bayonet defensive tactics lesson that several trainees had attempted, not to learn with him, but to actually bayonet him. At the next training session, Imi rectified this uncooperative attitude by sprawling his attacker with a kick, halting any further "tests." This incident prompted Imi to reinforce a proper student attitude: "Be humble." Proving oneself is not necessary. Humility and respect, Imi emphasized, prevent injury, losing face, or turning away from *krav maga* or any other demanding pursuit as a result of frustration. In 1964, after retiring as chief instructor, Imi began to adapt his system for civilian use. This civilian form of *krav maga* is the focus of this book.

In 1970 he began teaching a state-recognized *krav maga* instructor's course. He encouraged the instructors to join military, security, and police units or to establish themselves as professional instructors within the civilian community. Imi focused both on teaching professionals and adapting his system to provide ordinary civilians—men, women, and children—with solutions to avoid and/or end a violent encounter. In 1978 Imi, along with his senior students—including his successor, current Grandmaster Haim Gidon, established the *Ha Agudah L'Krav Maga Yisraeli* or the Israeli Krav Maga Association (IKMA) in his hometown, Netanya, to promote *krav maga* throughout the world for both civilians and the professional security community.

In 1979 Imi traveled to the United States with several English-speaking senior instructors to promote the *krav maga* system. The first international *krav maga* assistant instructor's course was held in 1981 in Netanya, Israel.

And now the story of *krav maga*'s lineage comes down to me. I trained for three years privately under senior instructor Rick Blitstein, and for one summer with senior instructor Alan Feldman. Rick eventually sent me to Grandmaster Gidon for instructor certification. I am honored to serve as Grandmaster Gidon's personal ambassador and lead instructor in the United States. The Grandmaster and his top instructors frequently visit my classes in New York and New Jersey to guest instruct. Former *krav maga* chief military instructor Boaz Aviram also occasionally co-teaches with me in New York City, as do Rick Blitstein and Alan Feldman. I typically visit Israel twice a year or more for advanced training.

About the IKMA Professional Committee

The Israeli Krav Maga Association (IKMA) Professional Committee assists Grandmaster Gidon. This professional committee includes some of the highest-ranking Israeli IKMA instructors, including Ohad Gidon, Yoav Krayn, and Yigal Arbiv.

Ohad Gidon   Sixth *dan,* he is one of the highest-ranking instructors in Israel. Ohad began his *krav maga* training under Imi and other senior IKMA instructors. Ohad is now instrumental in *krav maga*'s development and curriculum, along with his father, Grandmaster Gidon. Ohad is recognized as a "senior coach" by Wingate.

Yoav Krayn   Fourth *dan,* he is one of the highest-ranking instructors, having also trained with Imi and other senior instructors. Yoav has trained under Grandmaster Gidon since 1985 and serves as general secretary for the IKMA.

Yigal Arbiv   Third *dan,* he is one of Grandmaster Haim Gidon's top instructors. After serving in an elite paratroop unit as a weapons specialist, Yigal attended Wingate to receive his *krav maga* "senior coach's" certification. Yigal is a professional security specialist and *krav maga* instructor.

Ohad, Yoav, and Yigal regularly travel abroad to teach law-enforcement personnel as well as civilians. Each of these senior-level instructors has received numerous commendations from professional security agencies and accolades in the civilian sector.

Using Your Head

Imi was once asked why he did not commercialize black-belt training materials and charge a high fee. In response, Imi recalled a time he forced himself to learn a German poem verbatim, knowing in advance he would be tested in the next twenty minutes. He recited the poem, received a "Well done" from the teacher, and subsequently forgot the poem one minute later, for good. Rather than promote short-lived learning by rote, Imi emphasized developing a lasting ability. To accomplish this, he incorporated mental imagery into the training program. Your training comes from your mind absorbing, retaining, translating, and combining your instincts and learning and translating them into action. In *krav maga,* you will physically practice techniques over and over until they become second nature. You will also visualize executing those techniques in real situations.

The *krav maga* system, does not rely solely on defensive action to thwart an attack but also on a simultaneous (or as near as possible simultaneous) defense and attack. Merge your combatives into an overwhelming continuous attack; seamlessly and instinctively combining different combative techniques to keep your body in combat motion, the basis of *retzev* counterattacks.

Krav maga's combination of simultaneous defense and attack techniques underpin the system. Each technique is a building block in assembling a formidable self-defense foundation. The building blocks are cumulative and integrated. For example, the same technique can be used with slight modifications to defend yourself against a choke, a knife, or a gun held to your throat from the front. Even when faced with unfamiliar situations, the building blocks and theory underpinning them will likely present a solution. The integration of synchronized defensive and offensive techniques in a continuous flow, *retzev* counterattack is the backbone of the *krav maga* system. Only practice will help you to build *retzev* into your personal repertoire, molding you into a true *kravist.*

When faced with a hostile situation, you have a choice: fight or flight. I cannot overstate the importance of avoidance, retreat, and escape. Escape from a potential confrontation is usually the best option. Escape, however, is not always possible. When you cannot escape, you fight. The self-defense techniques you will soon learn will help you to repel or neutralize an attack, causing minimum injury to the attacker, but preserving the option of more debilitating counterattacks.

The Israel Defense Force, the Israel National Police, and the security agencies now train their personnel in *krav maga.* Such personnel use *krav maga* techniques nearly every day to safeguard personal weapons, defend against unarmed and armed attacks, apprehend suspects, and perform other security-related

---

Krav Maga's Belt-Ranking System ✦

To help separate the *krav maga* system into manageable learning segments for civilians, Imi created a belt-ranking system and focused the system on the most common types of unarmed street attacks. *Krav maga*'s self-defense phase includes the first four belt levels of yellow, orange, green, and blue, including more than one hundred joint-lock and choke-hold variations. In this book, you will learn techniques that correspond mostly to the first two belt levels: yellow and orange. After blue belt *krav maga* begins to emphasize advanced close-quarters-combat phases including weapon-against-weapon techniques. The most advanced black-belt levels focus on professional security and military applications along with teaching.

✦

activities. Since its inception, *krav maga* has helped to make the Israeli military one of the most respected and effective fighting forces in the world. As a result, the *krav maga* self-defense system continues to expand internationally, both among professionals and civilians. At the time of this writing, *krav maga* is taught in more than two dozen countries.

About Former Chief Military Instructor Boaz Aviram

Former chief military *krav maga* instructor Boaz Aviram received his advanced black-belt certification from Imi Lichtenfeld and served two years as the Israel Defense Forces' (IDF) chief instructor for combat fitness and close-quarters combat. As chief military *krav maga* instructor, Boaz oversaw and ran the entire *krav maga* instructor training course, including certifying other instructors and the IDF's elite units. Boaz is recognized as a "senior coach" by Wingate. Imi honored Boaz as one of *krav maga*'s top instructors and recognized his contributions to the *krav maga* system.

About Senior Instructor Rick Blitstein ⟵

Senior instructor Rick Blitstein is one of a few select individuals chosen in 1981 to attend the first international instructor's course in Netanya, Israel, under the watchful eye of *krav maga* founder and first Grandmaster Imi Lichtenfeld. Rick was taught for the purpose of introducing *krav maga* to the United States. He has taught civilians, professional security, and law enforcement personnel for more than two decades. Rick continues to teach and promote *krav maga* and continues to advance his knowledge under Grandmaster Gidon of the Israeli Krav Maga Association. Rick sent his student and close friend, David Kahn (the author of this book), to Grandmaster Gidon for advanced instructor certification.

⟵

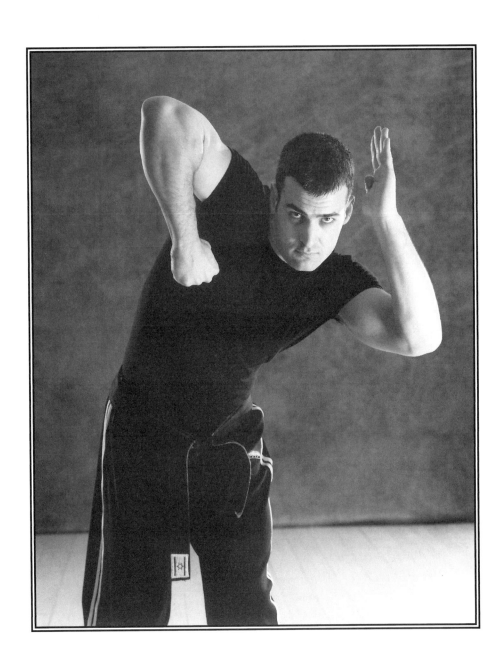

CHAPTER 2

The Philosophy Behind *Krav Maga*

Understand the six pillars of *krav maga* and you'll be well on your way to becoming a *kravist*

Krav maga will prepare you with the mind-set and physical skills you need to survive nearly any onslaught. You'll learn how to react with speed, economy of motion, and the appropriate measure of force. Indeed, in *krav maga*, you should never respond with more force than necessary.

The philosophy behind *krav maga* differs greatly from other types of martial arts and self-defense systems. Understanding the following philosophical pillars will help you to better absorb the training program—and understand why certain aspects of the training are needed. To become a successful *kravist*, you must master each of the following six components of the method:

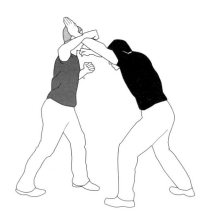

Simultaneous Defense and Attack Traditional close-quarters combat includes both offensive and defensive movements, and you must understand both to become a successful *kravist,* a term I have coined for someone accomplished in the *krav maga* system. At the same time, you must combine your defense and offense into one complete strategy. For example, if someone is choking you, not only will you remove his or her hands from your throat (a defensive movement), you will simultaneously counterattack to the eyes, groin, or throat (all offensive movements). If you merely reacted defensively by removing the attacker's hands, your attacker would simply move on to some other type of attack. You would find yourself locked in a never-ending series of defensive movements, and, at any moment, your attacker could gain the decisive advantage.

Continuous Motion   Unlike other types of martial arts, *krav maga* emphasizes *retzev,* a Hebrew word that means "continuous motion." To become a successful *kravist,* you must seamlessly integrate synchronized defensive and offensive techniques in an intuitive manner. It is imperative to understand the difference between *retzev* and merely a series of counterattacks. Whereas a series of attacks lacks continuity and does not flow automatically, *retzev* teaches you to move your body instinctively in combat motion without thinking about your next move. When in a dangerous situation, you'll automatically call upon your physical and mental training and launch a series of punches, kicks, grabs, and other moves. You'll move quickly and decisively—and your attacker will not have time to react.

Decisive Action   You must be both decisive and quick when you respond to a violent encounter. You also must put aside any apprehension about hurting your opponent. Although you may consider it unfair to stomp on an opponent's testicles or exposed neck, you cannot worry about fighting etiquette when your self-preservation is at stake. Street criminals, deranged individuals, or terrorists have made the decision to harm or murder. You cannot reason with these types of assailants or talk your way out of most dangerous situations. Note, however, that a street criminal might not always intend to inflict serious bodily harm or take your life, whereas a professionally trained killer or psychopath will have no such reservations. Although the force of your reaction is a judgment call, you will learn to read intentions and body language of an attacker and use force accordingly.

In *krav maga* you will learn to do whatever is necessary to overcome a dangerous threat, particularly if you feel your life is at stake. This may include multiple strikes to the groin, throat, and kidneys. You may need to poke your finger into an eye, shout into an attacker's ear, slam your forehead into someone's nose, or bite someone's neck. Because of this philosophy, *krav maga* is not suited for traditional sporting tournaments and must be practiced under controlled conditions. In short, controlled ferocity and brutality are a prerequisite to *krav maga* training. This is one reason why I recommend you seek a certified instructor to better absorb and employ the information you gain from reading this book.

A Focus on Vulnerable Soft Tissue and Pressure Points *Krav maga* is well known for its emphasis on counterattacking against soft tissue such as the groin, throat, and eyes. In chapter 3 you will learn how to strike or manipulate the body's most accessible pressure points to neutralize your opponent.

A Building Block Learning Process In *krav maga* you will learn one elemental technique and then build on it over time. You'll start with the simplest defenses, known as the the 360-degree instinctive defense, to enhance your peripheral vision and protect yourself from being hit from an outside attack. You'll then learn basic upper and lower body strikes—the art of using your fists, hands, elbows, knees, and feet to hit your attacker. You'll also learn how to defend against incoming strikes, tackles, chokes, and other movements. With more advanced training not included in this book, you will progress to more complex defenses, such as disarming an attacker who has a bladed weapon, firearm, hand grenade, and even rocks. *Krav maga* is world-renowned for these disarming techniques.

Krav maga has received international acclaim from security professionals and civilians alike for its practical techniques, which rely on instinctive body movements that can be performed under pressure, can be quickly learned and retained, and are based on building blocks that, when combined, are applicable to life-threatening situations.

Subduing Techniques The system also incorporates subduing techniques that may escalate or de-escalate a situation quickly. Such techniques may include, for example, the proper way to grab and, if necessary, break an opponent's finger to exert maximum control, and a myriad other joint locks, many of which are beyond the scope of this book.

Making Your Training as Real as Possible

Imi designed *krav maga* for people of all shapes, sizes, ages, and physical abilities. He once said, "I can teach you only as you are . . . [but] I will bring you to the highest level of what you are." Although he designed *krav maga* for soldiers, the techniques work just as well when used by civilians. *Krav maga*'s effectiveness does not rely on your physical prowess but, instead, on simple, combined movements. Imi liked to say, "Anybody can learn it. Anybody must learn it."

When you find yourself in a crisis situation, you'll automatically feel an explosive combination of adrenaline, fear, panic, and rage. *Krav maga* training will help you overcome the fight paralysis that can easily set in when such feelings and thoughts confront you. You'll learn how to alleviate fear, panic, and other sensations as you prepare your body and mind to take the proper course of action. You'll physically learn effective techniques while mentally adjusting to a harsh, violent reality. I suggest you practice the *krav maga* training methods in upcoming chapters while under extreme simulated pressure—in the most realistic setting possible—to develop the mental preparedness you need to react in life-threatening situations. It's one thing to go through the motions alone in your living room. It's quite another to practice the techniques with a partner who simulates a real attack. As you repeat techniques and situations at real speed (with safety in mind), you'll develop your fighting prowess. The *krav maga* techniques will become your automatic reflex whenever you find yourself in danger.

To best absorb the *krav maga* training, you must inject realism into your training. Imi recognized that actual violence differs greatly from choreographed training. All too often, martial artists who have devoted many years to training have found their skills inapplicable when faced with a trained or untrained opponent in an unpredictable, violent environment. To avoid freezing under pressure, you must train under pressure. For example, practice with a training partner or trusted friend to simulate attack situations using extreme control. Do the mock attacks and corresponding defenses at half-speed to stay safe and avoid injury. (I recommend learning these sparring techniques under a qualified instructor.) Only as you develop control and a working familiarity with a training partner can you begin to move at full speed. You must remember that the moves are designed to neutralize an attack at its inception. If practiced without caution or incorrectly, you could easily injure your training partner.

Visualization and Scenario Planning

In addition to practicing with a partner who is simulating an attack, you can also use your mind to train your body to automatically and instinctively react to danger. This is where visualization and scenario planning apply. Visualization and scenario planning will boost your confidence, reduce fear, improve your fighting technique, and help you cope with sudden hostile situations because you will have envisioned them beforehand.

In the final chapter of this book, you will learn how to envision a potential problem and then develop a series of solutions to solve it. When you visualize a new experience, you deposit a new conditioned response into your brain's memory bank. We perform routine tasks such as brushing our teeth easily because these tasks are just that—routine. They become routine by repetition. When you visualize possible situations and your reactions to them over and over again, your brain immediately recalls your reaction whenever you physically find yourself in such a situation, and you react accordingly.

Your brain does not distinguish between the actual tasks you physically perform and the ones you imagine or visualize. If you're unsure about this, think about the drop you felt in the pit of your stomach as you watched a film clip of a roller-coaster. Similarly, have you ever felt your hearting beating or palms sweating while watching a horror film? On one level you know that the film's serial killer is not actually in the room threatening your life. On another level, however, you don't.

Athletes have known about the power of visualization for many years and have used it with great success. Professional basketball players visualize themselves sinking a free throw before physically throwing the ball. Runners and swimmers imagine an entire event before stepping up to the starting line or pool edge. Golfers visualize their swing and "see" the ball travel where they want it to go. In each case, the mental rehearsal enhances the actual performance.

The Language of *Krav Maga*

Throughout this book the following terms will appear quite frequently. Once you understand the language of *krav maga,* you can better understand the method.

Danger Zone: Your danger zone is the range inside which someone can successfully reach you with their legs, arms, or a weapon.

***Glicha*:** You'll learn more about this sliding step in chapter 5. As with *secoul* (see below), *glicha* helps you make up ground and move in toward an attacker for a kick, shifting your body weight forward. Your base leg and entire body slides toward your attacker as you execute a kick, creating more impact.

***Kravist*:** I coined this term to describe anyone who is accomplished within the *krav maga* system, a fighter.

***Retzev*:** In Hebrew this word means "continuous motion," and it underpins the *krav maga* system. Rather than *thinking* about your defense and *then* executing it, you will train your mind and your body to seamlessly combine a series of strikes. When you master *retzev,* you react without thinking. You move continuously, with your punches seamlessly transitioning into elbow strikes, for example. Even though you may start out on the defensive, you will naturally, through *retzev,* move to the offensive or continuous combat motion. During *retzev,* you merge all of your *krav maga* training into an overwhelming continuous attack, instinctively combining numerous combatives.

Same side: Your same side arm or leg faces your opponent when you are opposite of one another. For example, if your right side is closest to your opponent's left side, your same side arm is your right arm.

***Secoul*:** This Hebrew word means "stepping sidekick." You'll learn how to use *secoul* in chapter 5. Basically, you step your rear foot toward your attacker, stepping behind your front kicking leg just before launching a kick. This helps you to cover ground and set up the proper distance for a kick while shifting your body weight into the kick.

You can do the same. By thinking about possible situations and seeing yourself reacting to them, you will be better prepared to summon the appropriate actions, even when your body has never before been put in that specific situation. For visualization to work effectively, you must envision a situation in great detail. Hear the noises, feel the vibrations, and see everything around you. This will help you mentally craft an accurate and thought-through response that you can file away. The more variations you file away, the better your chances of summoning a conditioned response when needed.

For example, imagine yourself sitting on a subway car. No one is sitting to your right or to your left. The subway car is sparsely occupied. You see an older man reading a paper at one end of the car and a mother and child at the opposite end of the car. Across from you, you see two teenage would-be toughs staring at you. The teen directly opposite you begins to stand up. He's clenching his fists.

Now visualize your reactions to the teen's possible modes of attack. Think about what you would do if he were to throw a straight punch with his right arm at your head. One option, if you are still seated, might be a swift powerful kick to his groin with your left leg while simultaneously bringing your arms up to defend your upper body. You then immediately stand up to kick him again in the groin, midsection, or face with your opposite leg and move behind him to his "deadside" or out of his direct line of sight. You'll more easily be able to visualize various offensive and defensive strategies once you learn the actual fighting techniques. For now, however, you have a good idea about why visualization and scenario planning is integral to your survival as a *kravist*.

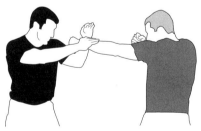

When facing your opponent's live side, you stand at a disadvantage.

Live Side　When you are facing the front of your opponent and your opponent can both see you and use all four arms and legs against you, you are facing his or her *live side*.

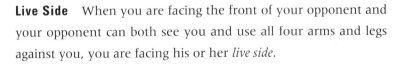

Dead Side   Your opponent's dead side, in contrast to his live side, places you behind his near shoulder or facing his back. You are in an advantageous position to counterattack and control him because it is difficult for him to use his arm and leg farthest away from you to attack you. You should always move to the dead side when possible. This also places the opponent between you and any additional third-party threat.

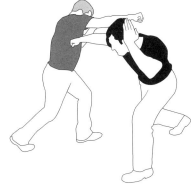

Always move to an attacker's dead side whenever possible.

Outside Defense   An outside defense, such as the 360-degree instinctive defense, counters an outside attack—that is, an attack directed at you from the outside of your body to the inside. A slap to the face or hook punch are examples of outside attacks.

Inside Defense   An inside defense, such as punch defense #1 in chapter 4, defends against an inside or straight attack involving thrusting motion, such as jabbing your finger into someone's eye or punching someone in the nose.

Underneath Defense   An underneath defense counters an upward attack, such as an uppercut punch or stab with an edged weapon to the navel.

Over-the-Top Attack   An over-the-top attack slams down on your opponent. Tactically, this type of strike can be used to overcome your opponent's defense. An over-the-top attack may involve hitting someone over the head with a stick or with an inverted elbow.

Krav Maga's Behavioral Code ⟶

Imi emphasized good citizenship and a strong sense of morality. The following pillars of Imi's system help summarize his teachings.

Good Citizenship   Treat your fellow citizens with respect and obey the law. Imi sought to instill "a sense of self-worth."

Train Properly to Avoid Injury   Do not injure your partner or yourself by training haphazardly or overaggressively.

Act Humbly   Do not show off your skills or provoke others to test your mettle. Act courteously toward others. As Imi said, "The most necessary thing is to educate you—and that is the hardest thing—to be humble. You must be so humble that you don't want to show him that you're better than him. That is one of the most necessary things for pupils. If a pupil tells me, 'I fought him and beat him,' it's no good."*

Avoid Confrontation   Avoid or de-escalate a potential violent situation whenever possible. When asked about a hypothetical confrontation that could be avoided, Imi responded, "Know what I told you—to be humble. I don't want to get beaten. I don't want to beat him. My purpose in learning *krav maga* is not to get hurt. If you beat him, you want to show him you can beat him. If you turn away, you have enough confidence."*

Do Not Use Unnecessary Force   Respond to a threat or attack with only the necessary amount of force to neutralize the attack. Imi underscored, "That is the most necessary and difficult thing in *krav maga*—that I must be so good that I don't have to kill." Imi also quipped, "Why do you want to break a dead man's arm?"*

⟶

*Excerpts from Imi Lichtenfeld's demonstration in Cleveland, Ohio, April 1984, courtesy of Rick Blitstein.

Legal Considerations

You must have a reasonable fear of harm to use physical force to defend yourself. If you inflict serious bodily harm or take another person's life, you must be legally justified. Only when you fear for your own life or that of another can you use lethal force. Under English common law, deadly force is never justifiable to protect property. For example, if someone keys your car, spits at you, or knocks over your mailbox, you may not resort to force to settle the score.

Reasonable force is best viewed on a sliding scale. The level of force employed is often dependent on an assailant's capability, opportunity, and intent. You can measure an attacker's capability in several ways. A weapon, large physical size, or displayed martial prowess, such as a fighting stance, all increase the assailant's measure of capability. American law, for example, generally recognizes a "disparity of force" when an attacker possesses recognizable physical advantages or prowess, such as significant height, strength, and weight, or trained fighting skills.

To assess the necessity of using force, you must look at several factors, including your opportunity to retreat. Retreat can be problematic if you are with another party such as a child or an elderly companion, or if you are in an enclosed area. Intent often involves the wielding of a weapon and verbal threats to your life and limb. When the threat is serious and imminent, a working knowledge of *krav maga* can mean the difference between successful self-defense and suffering harm.

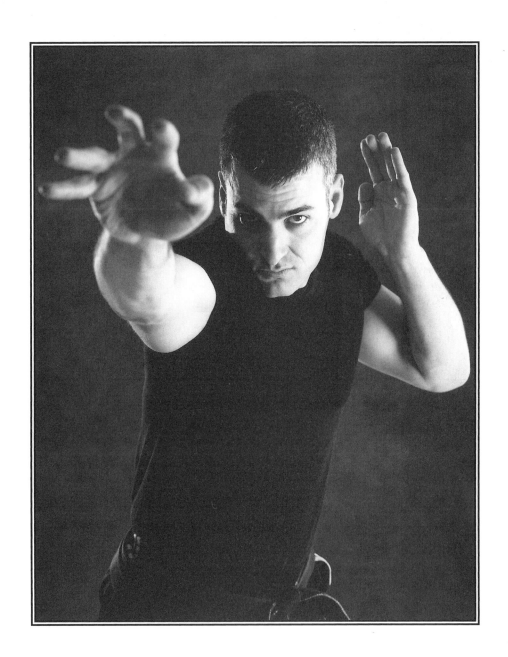

CHAPTER 3

The Mind of a *Kravist*

To react instinctively,
you must embody *krav maga*

If someone attempts to slap you in the face, there are two possible outcomes: you either get slapped or you avoid getting slapped. Many people, if they see the incoming slap in time, will stop it. Others, if they do see the slap, become paralyzed into inaction. *Krav maga* will help you avoid freezing under pressure. You'll learn how to use your intuitive reaction to defend yourself in any way you can. Even if you do not perform the preferred technique but still prevent the slap, you have done *krav maga*. *Krav maga* is whatever your body successfully does to save yourself from physical harm.

To make the method yours and react instinctively, you must put just as much emphasis on mental training as you do on the physical. In a physical confrontation, you may experience a combined surge of stress, fear, and excitement. When you are fearful, the nervous system increases the body's physical capabilities by injecting adrenaline into the bloodstream. Although fear helps you to survive by quickening your heart rate and sending more oxygenated blood to your muscles, you must harness your fear and remain levelheaded. Too much fear can make your legs quiver and creates the sensation of a lump in your throat. You must control these involuntary body responses to execute the correct self-defense reactions. You will need both physical and mental training to learn how to react to this fear-induced adrenaline rush.

In short, mental and physical conditioning allows you to harness your adrenaline and channel it into action. Mental confidence and toughness, in particular, provides a decisive advantage in a violent encounter. When you feel confident, you believe that your training will carry the day regardless of an opponent's physical size, possession of a weapon, or his gang of buddies backing him up. Confidence, however, must not lead to overconfidence. *Do not underestimate your opponent, and always expect the unexpected.* Mental conditioning will help build your confidence, preventing the panic that can lead to freezing or poor decision making. Mental conditioning will also allow you to de-escalate or walk away (always the best solution if possible) from a potentially violent situation.

Throughout the *krav maga* training program, you'll learn numerous ways to hone your mental skills. With proper training, you'll learn how to use fear and other negative emotions to your advantage. You'll harness the energy and power from your body's fight-or-flight response rather than freezing under pressure. Conversely, if you merely read through this book but don't actually train on a regular basis, the physical trauma, coupled with fright and shock, will most likely negate rational thought and paralyze you into inaction. When in danger, the brain searches its records for a response. In a fight, if an opponent takes an unanticipated or unrecognized action, the brain cannot find a practiced response, resulting in decision paralysis.

Denial is the most common obstacle to taking appropriate action. Often, with an untrained mind and body, it's tough to process or accept that someone else poses imminent danger to life and limb. A victim may wonder, "Why would a stranger attack me?" This thinking may continue, for example, even after the third, fourth, or fifth stab wound.

This is why you must hone your mental and physical skills until you can call on them without thinking. With enough practice, you'll train your muscles to react instinctively and swiftly. Only proper training can trigger this fighting response.

The Four Steps to Action

When confronted with the threat of violence, the mind goes through a series of steps to choose a response. These reaction stages include the following:

1. **Threat recognition.** In analyzing a potential violent situation, the mind must recognize the danger and then process it.
2. **Situation analysis.** Once the mind recognizes the danger, it contemplates the possible outcomes and takes in any additional clues that may be helpful in arriving at a choice of action.
3. **Choice of action.** After processing the danger's potential outcome or outcomes, the mind quickly considers available courses of action and chooses one. This leads to the final stage, action or inaction.
4. **Action or inaction.** After the mind settles on a reaction, it propels the body into action—or the paralysis of inaction.

Training improves this reaction flow by allowing you to quickly assess violent situations. Training ingrains the appropriate responses into your memory. Whether the threat comes from a punch, choke, knife, or gun, you will already know how to react. Training will improve your physical reaction time. Equally important, it will speed your ability to choose the most suitable technique for a given situation.

To react instinctively, you must train both your mind and your body. Despite the best mental training, the heat of the moment can inhibit your optimum response. Therefore you need physical training as well. In *krav maga* you will learn a few elementary techniques that you can perform instinctively and apply to a wide variety of situations. You'll learn how to protect your vital points and organs. Equally important, you'll know how to debilitate an opponent by striking his or her vital points and organs. If the situation requires it, *krav maga* will teach you how to maximize the damage you can inflict by striking, kneeing, kicking, chopping, gouging, choking, dislocating joints, breaking bones, and taking your opponent down to the ground.

Reacting to an Attack

An attack launched by surprise will force you to react from an unprepared state. Therefore your self-defense reaction must be instinctive and reflexive. *Krav maga* training prepares you for just that. Your subconscious mind will turn your instinctive trained responses into immediate action. Instinct assumes control, for example, in deflecting an incoming straight punch with whichever of your hands is best positioned. Alternatively, you might use a body defense by moving your head away from the blow while tucking your chin. The same instincts will condition you to use your front leg to deflect a straight kick targeting your groin. Practicing and repeating techniques will embed them in your consciousness so you can summon them in a moment of need.

One of the most effective lessons *krav maga* can teach you, however, is to not to be taken by surprise in the first place. Once you develop an awareness of your environment—any environment—you'll notice at all times who and what surrounds you. By recognizing a potential threat before it actually becomes a threat, you can avoid a potentially hazardous situation. The best defense against any attack is removing yourself from the situation before the attack can take place. Only awareness of your environment can help you do that. In an unknown environment, keep your head subtly swiveling by shifting your eye movements, using your peripheral vision, and panning for potential threats. Constantly survey your surroundings.

For example, if you notice a questionable group of young men congregating on the street corner in the direction you are walking, you can avoid a confrontation by walking on the opposite side of the street. Here's another example. Let's say you are walking down the street and you sense that someone is following you. If there is enough distance, you might pretend to check the back of your shoe or pants leg. This will give you an opportunity to to steal a look behind you to see who is there. Check out the person behind you without shooting an emotional look over your shoulder. An emotional look will tell the potential assailant that you are aware of his presence and suspect his intentions, which isn't something you necessarily want. If you deliver a body language message of, "I will not be a victim," you'll meet the potential threat head-on. Although such deterrent behavior may thwart a potential attack, it runs the risk of escalating a situation when dealing with an adversary primed for a confrontation.

Let's take a look at a third example. Let's say you are walking down the street and notice a deranged or otherwise threatening person behind or near you in close proximity. What do you do? You could accelerate your pace to gain distance or you could move laterally to let the person pass and keep the threat in front of you. The latter is usually the better option.

Finally, let's say you are watching a potential adversary's hand movements. You notice that his hands are hidden in a pocket but sense that the adversary is about to pull out a weapon. Along the same lines, recognition of a bulge on a potential assailant's body—a possible weapon—will allow you to take the initiative.

Understanding the Human Body

The human body can withstand a high amount of physical punishment. To be sure, certain attacks can be lethal; but even when severely injured, the body can perform miraculous feats. Adrenaline is a powerful energizer and allows the body to momentarily insulate itself against pain. The body's resilience works for both

Twenty-four Vulnerable Targets

In *krav maga* you learn to avoid hard skeletal bones such as the crown of the skull and focus your efforts on easy-to-strike soft tissues. During a confrontation, you also want to protect these areas from incoming strikes. Attack the most vulnerable areas (eyes, neck, temples) only when you feel your life is in danger. Vulnerable targets include.*

1. Hair
2. Eyes
3. Temples
4. Base of the skull
5. Nose
6. Ears
7. Mouth
8. Chin and jaw
9. Throat (specifically the windpipe)
10. Sides, back, and hollow of the neck
11. Base of the neck
12. Clavicles
13. Elbows
14. Ribs
15. Solar plexus
16. Back and kidneys
17. Stomach
18. Fingers
19. Testicles
20. Thighs
21. Knees
22. Skin
23. Ankles
24. Top of the feet

* Ben-Asher, Col. David. *Fighting Fit, the Israel Defense Forces Guide to Physical Fitness and Self-Defense.* Perigree Books (1983).

victim and assailant. Note that an assailant under the influence of drugs may acquire yet another layer of pain insulation and artificially increased strength.

Krav maga will give you the advantage in any threatening situation. To stop an assailant, *krav maga* primarily targets the body's vital soft tissue, chiefly the groin, neck, and eyes. Other secondary targets include the kidneys, solar plexus, knees, liver, joints, fingers, nerve centers, and other smaller fragile bones. *Krav maga* differs from other self-defense systems that may rely primarily on targeting difficult to locate nerve centers. In the heat of a struggle, this type of precise combative is extremely difficult. Conversely, a *krav maga* combative to the groin is precise enough to debilitate the opponent and is simple to deliver.

Let's take a closer look at how you will strike at and use vulnerable sections of your opponent's body during a confrontation, starting at the top of the body and working down to the feet.

Hair   You can grip your opponent's hair to immobilize the head or expose the throat for attack. You can do so by sliding one hand through the hair with the fingers wide apart. Once the hair is between the spread fingers, close your hand into a tight fist and forcefully pull at the scalp to create a strong grip and inflict significant pain. Yank longer hair, especially when in a ponytail, in one direction or another to set up a throat strike or to damage the neck.

Eyes   A light finger whip to the eye can cause watering and temporary blinding. A thrusting attack with a finger can crush an eyeball or dislodge it from its socket. In addition to intense pain, blinding an assailant provides easier access for other attacks and allows you to get away. Because strikes to the eyes can be fatal, only use them if the threat warrants this type of defense.

Temples   Just above your jaw joint, the temples form the thinnest part of the skull and house a sensitive nerve center. Because the brain is the least protected by the skull at the temples, a strike here can produce hemorrhaging. Deliver a strike to the temple with a protruding knuckle or pointlike weapon of opportunity such as a cell phone or pen. As noted with eye strikes, a temple strike can be fatal and should only be used as a last resort.

Base of the Skull Striking here can create shock, concussion, paralysis, or death because the brain stem is located here.

The Nose The nose is extremely fragile and may be attacked with a number of strikes including punches, hammer fists, ridge hand, palm heel, elbows, and head butts. (You'll learn more about such strikes in upcoming chapters.) You can easily break the nose with a high kick to the face or an upper body strike while an opponent is standing or on the ground. Breaking an opponent's nose can be debilitating, but a determined attacker can continue to fight despite the pain, blood, and watery eyes. You can also lift the nose (filtrum) at the nostrils to pull or push the head back to create separation from an assailant or expose the throat to further strikes. A strike to the nose, depending on the angle, can also be lethal.

The Ears Boxing the ears will stun an opponent by throwing off the ear's inner equilibrium. A concussion from an eardrum rupture results when the large inner canal suffers trauma. Located behind the ear is the mastoid (jaw bone) that, when struck hard, disrupts the opponent's equilibrium.

The Chin, Jaw, and Mouth A blow to the chin can disorient an opponent by literally shaking the brain. A chin or jaw strike may result in a knockout by rattling the brain against the skull wall and producing localized brain damage. In addition, the jaw is flush with nerve centers that are vulnerable to punches, palm heels, elbows, or a head-level kick. The mouth is vulnerable to these types of attacks, too, but keep in mind that a mouth strike is likely to hit the teeth. By their nature, the teeth are sharp and can damage your fist, risking infection and blood poisoning.

The Throat   A punch, chop, or other strike to the throat can cause severe damage or death. In addition, strangulation can result in a loss of consciousness or death. You can grab and squeeze the wind pipe to deprive the brain of oxygen or crush it by a strike. Only attack this target during a life-threatening confrontation.

The Sides and Back of the Neck   You can target the sides of the neck with "blood chokes." This compresses the carotid artery in the neck that supplies oxygen to the brain. If you restrict blood flow with a stranglehold, your assailant will lose consciousness in a few seconds. This type of hold differs from a stranglehold to the throat, which restricts air passage through the windpipe and may take longer to render an opponent unconscious. Prolonged constriction of the blood vessels and cutting off of breathing can also result in death.

Clavicles   A sharp blow here can break the clavicle, preventing your assailant from using his arms. You can also insert your fingers into the hollow between the bones and yank down forcefully to break the clavicle.

The Ribs   These bones form a protective yet fragile cage around the lungs. A sharp blow such as punch, kick, or knee can break the ribs, especially the floating ribs that have no direct attachment to the sternum. Broken ribs are extremely painful, and if a rib is broken with enough force it can puncture a lung.

Small of the Back   The central nerves of the body branch out from the base of the spine close to the surface of the small of the back.

The Kidneys   Located just above the small of the back, the kidneys are susceptible to damage from a blow such as a punch, chop, knee, or kick. In addition to acute pain, kidney failure may result.

The Solar Plexus   You can strike centrally above the naval and below the sternum to damage the liver or rupture the gall bladder, resulting in severe internal bleeding.

The Testicles   As you may already know, the testicles are a particularly vulnerable part of a male's anatomy, making them an obvious target for kicks, knees, and hand strikes. A strong blow to this area will result in debilitating pain and could damage the urinary bladder, resulting in internal bleeding or a fatal blood clot. Although a groin strike is one the most effective combatives, an opponent can experience a significant adrenaline surge before the pain registers and still continue an attack.

The Vulva   The female vulva is also highly sensitive to any kind of strike and, similarly, will cause significant pain.

The Knees, Elbows, and Other Joints   You can dislocate and fracture almost any joint in the body with a sharp blow or forceful countermovement against the joint's natural articulation. You can also manipulate joints to subdue your attacker.

The Thigh, Shin, and Foot   The top of the foot is especially vulnerable to a stomp with the heel, which may fracture many of the small bones. You can twist or break an ankle with a downward stomp, especially if the opponent is perched on the ball of his foot and the stomp is delivered to the Achilles tendon.

As you read through the body's vulnerable targets, you may have felt a bit uneasy. It may be difficult to read through a list of potential harms to another human, but you must remember that this person intends to harm you. You must do whatever is necessary to neutralize the threat. Hopefully, none of these counterattacks will ever be necessary, but this list of twenty-four targets should further remind you why *krav maga* emphasizes avoiding confrontation as your most important line of defense.

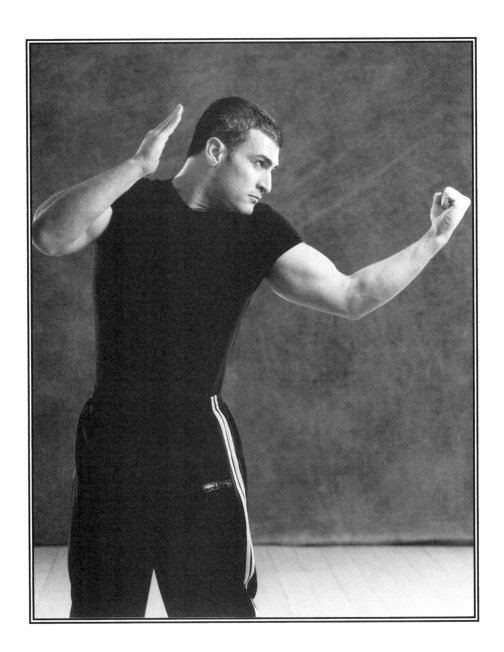

CHAPTER 4

Mastering Upper-Body Strikes

⌐

The power behind the punch comes from precise execution, not from body size or muscular strength

Many people think of hand-to-hand combat as exactly that: using your fists to strike at an opponent. Yet *krav maga* teaches you to use any and every part of your body—from the head to the foot—as tools to deliver strikes. Later in this book, you will learn how to use your knees, feet, forehead, and other body parts to defend yourself. In this chapter we'll begin with upper body strikes and defenses, teaching you how to use your fists, hands, and elbows to strike at your opponent. You'll build the top half of your *krav maga* technique arsenal first, along with the confidence to go with it.

These techniques are easy to learn, and work well when fighting at an intermediate distance. In coming chapters you'll learn additional techniques that will help you defend yourself at long-range and short-range distances. Then in chapter 9, you'll learn how to put everything you've learned together into a comprehensive training program that not only will help you to grow into a true *kravist*, but also will get you in the best shape of your life.

The Force Is with You

No matter your body size or muscular strength, you can deliver powerful strikes with your hands and elbows. When performing *krav maga* demonstrations in front of a crowd, I often illustrate this point by asking a large member from the audience—often a tall man who weighs in excess of two hundred pounds—to hold a protective pad. I then ask one of my instructors who is just five feet tall and about one hundred pounds to elbow the pad. Without fail, Elizabeth's powerful elbow will jolt the man. As you can see, you don't need a lot of body strength to punch and strike effectively. Precise execution of a punch or elbow strike will generate much more impact than muscling your way through one.

Physics teaches us that acceleration times mass equals force. In other words, your strike will generate more force if you accelerate your speed as you extend your arm and put all of your body weight (mass) behind your punch. This requires proper body positioning and technique. As I mentioned in chapter 1, *krav maga* techniques do not rely on strength. Rather, the system works for everyone of all shapes and sizes. A ninety-pound woman can easily incapacitate a 250-pound man if she puts all of her weight behind her strike and aims for a vulnerable target, such as the groin or throat.

Proper technique starts with a strong stance. In *krav maga* you will learn two basic stances from which to practice the techniques:

1. The regular left-outlet fighting stance
2. The regular right-outlet fighting stance

Although each exercise in this book teaches you in the left-outlet position, practice the techniques from the right-outlet stance as well, so you are comfortable fighting from both sides of your body. Both stances use the same leg and arm positioning. The difference between them is that in one, you place your left foot forward, and, into the other, you place your right foot forward. Your outlet stance protects your groin from incoming strikes and gives you a strong base of support to launch defensive and offensive movements with your arms or legs. Launch all of your strikes from this stance. From this position, you can easily kick with either your front or rear leg.

The Regular-Outlet Stance

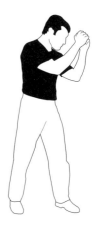

Place your feet close together with your toes facing forward. Rotate your toes clockwise as you turn your body 30 degrees to your right, coming into a left regular-outlet stance with your left arm and left leg forward. (You can also turn 30 degrees to your right to come into a right-regular-outlet stance, so that your right leg and arm are forward.) For the left outlet stance, take a step back with the right foot until you feel comfortable and balanced. Your feet should be about a shoulder width apart. While keeping the ball of your your right foot firmly planted, raise your back heel slightly and drop your body weight onto the ball of your foot. Allow just enough separation between your rear heel and the ground to slide a piece of paper under your foot. Your feet should be parallel and about 55 percent of your weight distributed over your front leg.

Position your arms in front of your face and slightly forward. Extend your arms so your upper arms are about parallel to the ground. Bend your elbows to form a 60-degree angle between your forearms and your upper arms. Hold your hands at eyebrow level, about six inches apart, but do not block your line of sight. For some trainees, especially those with large shoulders, this hand positioning can be uncomfortable. In this case position the width of your hands as you feel comfortable, but try to keep them within the width of your shoulders and your elbows close to your body. Cup your hands with the fingers held together. Tuck your chin and look up toward your imaginary opponent. In a real fighting situation, you will focus on his face as you retain an overall picture of his movements, especially his hands and legs.

From this stance you can move forward, laterally, and backward. Practice your footwork and move in all directions. Your feet should always move in concert. Do not overextend yourself. Practice switching from a left regular-outlet stance with your left leg forward to a right-regular-outlet stance, with your right leg forward. For example, from the left-outlet stance a rear kick with the right foot will bring you forward into a right-outlet stance. As you switch from one stance to another, keep your arms raised in your protective position. As your training progresses you will be able to seamlessly move from one stance into another.

You may wish to stand in a modified-outlet stance if you are concerned that someone near you may pose a threat. Keeping your hands in front of you at sternum level, cupped in front of you as if you were wringing your hands, will not escalate the situation by signaling a provocative movement or fighting position.

The Passive-Outlet Stance

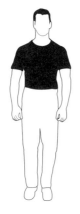

When possible, stand in your regular-outlet stance at all times during a confrontation. At times, however, you may be caught by surprise while you are standing in a passive-outlet stance. Most people do not stand in a regular-outlet stance but, rather, in a passive-outlet stance when not expecting confrontation. In the passive-outlet stance, your feet are under your hips and your arms are at your sides. Although this stance is not a strong fighting stance, you should practice delivering strikes from this stance and moving from your passive outlet into a regular outlet in the event you are caught by surprise.

The 360-Degree Instinctive Defense

Your 360-degree defenses counter outside attacks, such as slaps and roundhouse or hook punches, outside straight or sucker punches, in which an assailant attempts to punch you in the face from an indirect off angle out of your line of vision or knife and edged-weapon attacks.

The defense consists of seven movements.

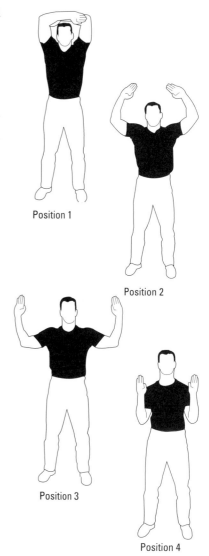

Position 1

Position 2

Position 3

Position 4

Position 1. Raise your arms overhead, crossing your forearms and forming a triangle with your arms. This arm position forms a protective shield around the top and sides of your head from attacks coming down toward your head.

Position 2. With your elbows still bent at 90-degree angles, lower your upper arms until they are 45 degrees from the ground and rotated slightly outward with your palms facing out. This protects you against unexpected attacks to the head.

Position 3. From position 2, lower your forearms to chest level, with your palms facing slightly out. If you thrust your arms outward from this position, opening your forearms to the sides, you can defend against such attacks as a hook or roundhouse punch, slap, and roundhouse kick to head.

Position 4. Draw your elbows against your sides with your fingertips facing up and the backs of your hands just in front of your shoulders to defend against a blow to the ribs or midsection.

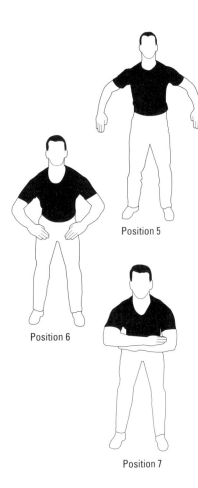

Position 5

Position 6

Position 7

Position 5. With your arms bent at 90-degree angles, lower your fingertips toward the ground with your palms facing back. Draw your elbows back, until your biceps (the muscle along the front of the upper arm) are parallel to the floor. This posture can help you defend against a knife attack.

Position 6. Bend your elbows in 45-degree angles and bring your hands in front of your hips with your elbows out to the sides. Bend forward slightly from the hips. This posture can help you defend against a knife attack.

Position 7. From position 6, place one forearm on top of the other, with your arms bent at 90-degree angles and your elbows out to the sides. Lean forward. Move your hips as far back as possible to guard your body from an incoming attack. This posture will help you to defend against a blade or pointed weapon.

Practice the 360-degree defenses as a seamless, modified circular movement, moving from one position into the next over and over again until the defenses become second nature. From start to finish, your path of movement and range of motion should resemble a circle.

How to Throw a Punch

The bones in your hand are small and fragile. If you don't use proper alignment, you can easily break them if you strike against hard bone. To make a fist, curl your fingers into your palms, placing your thumbs on top of your index fingers, not inside of your fist. Keep the back of your hand in line with your wrist and forearm. Any bend other than a slight downward angle of the wrist can cause serious damage, especially a rotation to the left or right, which takes the wrist out of its natural alignment. Hitting a target with your hands misaligned with your forearms can break the bones in your wrist. Aim for soft tissue targets whenever possible, lock your wrist, and make contact with the first two knuckles. To strengthen your wrists and knuckles for punching, do push-ups on your knuckles.

No matter what type of punch you deliver, shift your body weight through your strike. This allows you to place all of your body weight behind the punch, connecting with maximum force. When practicing punching, do not lock your elbows. Elbow injuries are often caused by punching powerfully without resistance. If the punch does not make contact, the ulna bone in the lower arm jams into the humerous bone in the upper arm. When not making contact with a training pad (or sparring partner), extend your arms about 90 percent as you deliver a strike. Strong pad and bag work will accustom your striking limbs to impact while building strength and stamina. Heavy bags are particularly useful for this type of training.

Here are some pointers for striking effectively.

Use your entire body   As you strike, move the entire body in concert. Rather than striking with only your hand or elbow, use your entire torso. As you propel all of your strength and body weight through the strike, you'll maximize your strike's impact.

Breathe   Exhale as you deliver the strike. Some people like to use a blood-curdling cry as they strike. Either technique—the cry or exhale—will prepare your body for both delivering a strike and receiving a strike. Exhaling facilitates oxygen transfer to your muscles, tempers your movements to keep you in control, and creates a vacuum to defend against a counterstrike.

Aim for Vulnerable Targets   You'll maximize your effort if you strike at the vulnerable targets mentioned in chapter 3, striking

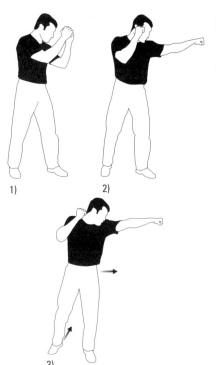

1) 2)

3)

at the most vulnerable targets only when the threat requires. Aiming for the body's soft tissues—the neck, groin, and other sensitive areas—helps increase the effectiveness of your strike.

The Straight Front Punch

When using this direct and fast strike, aim for the nose, jaw, or throat.

Stand in the left-outlet stance with your hands in loose fists. Step forward with your left foot and quickly draw your rear heel slightly in and back, thrusting your left hip into the strike. You are not jumping at the same time with both feet. There is an ever so brief pause between the steps as your entire body launches forward. Simultaneously extend your left arm, thrusting your fist toward your target, blading your body for maximum extension. As your arm extends to deliver the punch, tighten your fist, extending your entire body toward the target. Make contact with your hand parallel to the ground. Tuck your chin to protect your jaw and neck. After striking, return to your left-outlet stance.

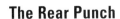

1) 2)

3)

The Rear Punch

Similar to the front punch, this technique best targets the nose, jaw, or throat.

Stand in the left-outlet stance with your hands in loose fists. Pivot your right leg slightly onto the ball of the foot as you drive your hips, rear shoulder, and arm forward toward your target, maximally extending your entire body into the strike. Tuck your chin into your right shoulder to protect it from an incoming strike.

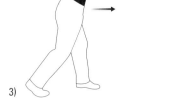

Creating a Punching Sequence

You can combine the front and rear punches into a highly effective (left/right) combination. Lead with the front punch, as it will reach the target more quickly than your rear. Withdraw the punching arm quickly into your fighting stance to maintain your defensive and offensive capability. As soon as you land the front punch and are retracting your arm, launch your rear punch. The momentum of drawing the front punch back will help draw the rear punch forward, creating greater impact.

If you must retreat, you can still sting your attacker. As you shuffle backward, launch a front punch to keep an oncoming attacker at bay. Retreat with the rear foot, followed by the front foot as the front arm simultaneously extends to punch.

The Short, Inverted Punch

This quick punch allows you to cover a short distance to close on your opponent.

Stand in a left-outlet stance with your hands in loose fists. Punch as if you were connecting with a front punch, except keep your pinky side of the hand facing the ground. The short, inverted punch differs from the straight punch because the knuckles are now vertical toward your target and the punching arm's elbow is close the body. Use the short, inverted punch to move inside while executing a defense against an outside (360-degree position 3, page 57) roundhouse ("hook") or slashlike movement. Your body explodes forward with a simultaneous defense and attack.

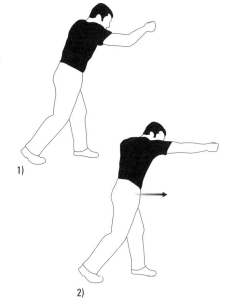

1)

2)

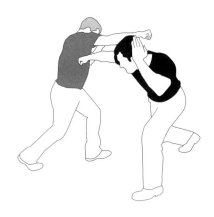

Low Defensive Punch

This low punch helps you defend against a strike to your head.

Stand in a left-outlet stance with your hands in loose fists. Perform the same movement as a front punch, except this time bend your knees, take a step out, and crouch low, aiming for the midsection or groin.

The Palm-Heel Strike

Similar to straight punches in footwork, weight redistribution, and chin positioning, the palm-heel strike is an effective intermediate-range strike, particularly for those who are not confident in the strength of their wrists and fists to execute regular punches.

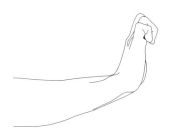

Starting from your regular-oulet stance, make a palm heel by tightly curling your fingers and pressing your thumb close to your hand. Bend your fingers toward your shoulder, exposing

---

Upper Body Drills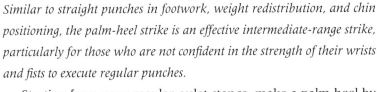

Using a heavy bag, sparring partner, or mirror, practice the following combinations. To familiarize yourself with various techniques, use the same drill but substitute the technique you wish to practice for the straight punches or palm heels.

1. From the left-outlet stance: 20 left-forward straight punches and 20 right-rear straight punches (or palm-heel strikes). Repeat the drill from the right-outlet stance, substituting the right forward arm.
2. Repeat the drill from the right-outlet stance: 20 straight right/left combinations with step and pivot.

your palm. Your knuckles should be facing upward. Throw a front punch with your hand in the palm-heel position, connecting with the heel of your hand.

The Front Roundhouse ("Hook") Punch

Roundhouse punches can circumvent or go around your opponent's defense. The punch's path follows whatever opening your opponent gives you. Targets usually include the jaw, cheek, throat, and ear. A note of caution: The mastoid behind the ear is dense bone and this target can damage your hand.

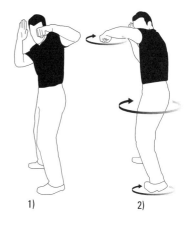

Begin in your regular-outlet stance with your hands protecting your face. Connect with your target with your front arm parallel to the ground with the elbow bent at 90 degrees. Make contact with the first two knuckles, your palm facing the ground. As you deliver the hook, pivot on your front foot in the same direction as the punch so that your front heel nearly faces your target. As you pivot your heel, turn the rest of your body, but keep your eyes on the target. Adjust your rear foot slightly to accommodate your front foot's movement. Keep your rear hand up in a fighting position.

The Rear Roundhouse Punch

This strike is similar to the front roundhouse, but you'll deliver it with your rear arm.

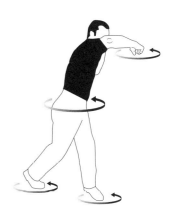

Begin in your regular-outlet stance with your hands protecting your face. As you deliver a roundhouse punch with your rear fist, pivot your rear in the same direction as the punch. This will increase the power of the strike. At the same time move the front

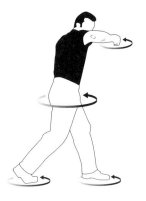

foot in the same direction to accommodate the rear foot's movement. Keep your chin tucked.

You can also try punching with your pinky down and thumb up. Although physiology dictates that you'll punch with less power because your deltoids and other shoulder muscles are not as actively involved, some practitioners prefer the "knuckles up" roundhouse punch because the movement feels more natural to them. In addition this hand position offers some additional protection to your exposed ribs.

The Front/Rear Roundhouse-Punch Combination

This one-two combination works well together and takes advantage of the momentum of your body.

Begin in your regular-outlet stance with your hands protecting your face. Deliver a front roundhouse strike. Then immediately follow up with a rear roundhouse punch.

The Roundhouse Body Shot

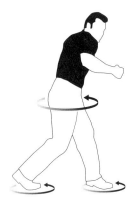

This technique delivers a roundhouse punch to the torso.

Perform the same lower body and hip movements as the high-front and -rear roundhouses, but change your hand position into an inverted punch, keeping your elbow in close to your torso and your forearm parallel to the ground. You can combine high and low roundhouse punches to form a devastating attack. Follow up with a high-front punch and then a low-rear punch or vice versa. In addition, you can throw a high/low or low/high combination with the same side arm.

Combination-Punch Drill

This drill combines straight punches with your roundhouse punches. This combination is highly effective and is a good foundation to begin *retzev* upper-body combatives.

1. From the left-outlet stance: 20 left/right straight punches and left/right roundhouse combinations. From the right-outlet stance: 20 right/left straight punches and right/left roundhouse combinations.
2. From the left-outlet stance: 20 left straight punches and left roundhouse combinations using the same arm. From the right-outlet stance: 20 right straight punches and right roundhouse combinations using the same arm.
3. From the left-outlet stance: 20 left-right straight combinational punches followed by 20 left-right roundhouse punches. From the right-outlet stance: 20 right-left straight combinational punches followed by 20 right-left roundhouse combinations.
4. From both the left- and right-outlet stances, create and vary combinations as you feel comfortable. Thinking through different combinations will help you master the techniques and build the base for *retzev*.

Body-"Shot" Straight Punches

This technique knocks the wind out of an opponent or, if delivered with enough force and accuracy, can break an opponent's ribs and damage internal organs. There are two types of body shot punches.

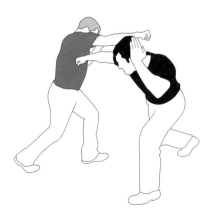

Body-shot punch 1. Bend your knees, bringing your upper body forward. You are in a modified crouch and should feel comfortable pivoting and stepping through to punch. The body movement is similar to your regular straight punches, but you'll execute the punch from a defensive crouch while stepping out that takes you out of the line of fire.

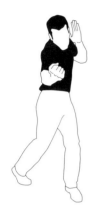

Body-shot punch 2. Deliver this punch with your forearm parallel to the ground, reaching up and in to your opponent. As you deliver this strike, move your lower body and hips in a modified pivoting movement. Practice this strike carefully because of the wrist's precarious position if not aligned properly. Targets will vary depending on your angle, height, and position and can include the groin, stomach, ribs, kidneys, and liver. Keep in mind that while body punches are effective, knees also provide one of the quickest methods to take an opponent down, as you will learn in chapter 5.

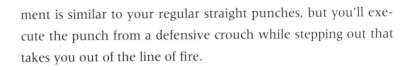

Using Elongated Weapons for Thrusting Strikes

Your synchronized lower- and upper-body movements will form the base for strikes with elongated blunt and edged weapons, such as the tip of a long umbrella.

Stand in your left-outlet stance. Grasp your weapon with your front hand. Thrust your weapon at your target as you would a front punch, stepping forward with your front leg and then following through with your rear leg. You'll learn how to use additional weapons of opportunity on page 75.

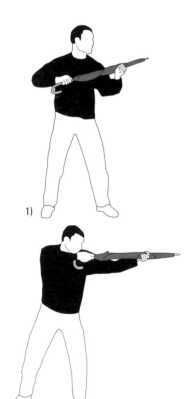

1)

2)

Body Defenses, Movement, and Absorption Against Punches

No matter how much you train with defenses, when you're faced with a determined attacker there is a good chance you will still get hit. Therefore you must train your body to move with and absorb strikes. When receiving a blow to the head, move your head in the direction of the strike. Do not tense and strengthen your neck to meet or resist the strike. This will only increase the strike's impact.

To understand why you should move in the direction of the strike, try this simple experiment. Hold out one of your hands and slap it full force with other hand. As you slap your hand, strengthen your outstretched arm and hold it tight on impact. Notice how the impact feels. Then, slap your hand again, but, this time, keep your outstretched arm loose on impact. You will feel much less impact as the loosened arm moves with the strike. The same will happen with your head when it moves with the strike, either to the side or backward. Practice moving and absorbing light open-handed strikes protecting your head with your hands with a trusted partner using minimum force. Don't allow your tongue to jut between your teeth, or you will accidentally bite it.

To better absorb body shots to your torso, you must create a vacuum by exhaling and strengthening your abdominal muscles. By exhaling on impact, you will literally avoid having the wind knocked out of you. In addition, tensing your midsection allows you to better withstand the strike. Try moving and absorbing your partner's light, controlled strikes with your eyes closed to make these drills more instinctive. Ask your partner to strike lightly at your torso as you practice moving with the strike, tightening your abdomen, and exhaling.

Krav Maga also employs many other body defenses that can help you to dodge or reduce the impact of strikes. They include the following:

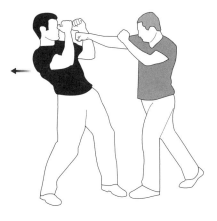

- **The upper-body retreat.** As the strike comes in, bend backward with your hands up. Hold your arms in the same position as in your outlet stance as you lean back from the hips and shift your body weight backward, away from the blow. Similarly, you can also move your body to the left or to the right.

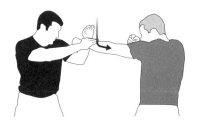

~ **Ducking.** As the strike comes in, bend your knees while keeping your body positioned in your outlet stance. Boxers are skilled in these weaving and bobbing movements. Note that bobbing and weaving exposes you to a knee attack to the head.

Inside Punch Defense 1

This is the more instinctive of the two inside-punch defenses you will learn. Inside-punch defense 1 is effective against the left/right combination that you learned previously. If you are standing directly opposite your opponent, nose to nose, your left arm will be aligned with his right arm and his left arm will be aligned with your right arm. You will use this defense to intercept and redirect the incoming punch.

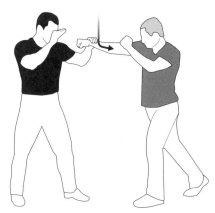

Stand in your regular-outlet stance. Position your fingers either in a palm heel or cupped as you would in your regular-outlet stance. As the punch comes in, use your arm on the same side (so if the punch is with the right arm, use your left arm) to redirect it with your palm, to the inside of your body. If possible, also move your head slightly opposite to deflect the direction of the punch and further ensure your safety. As you redirect the punch, you can move inward toward your opponent and simultaneously strike to the face with your other arm. Or you can stand your ground and follow up with a long-distance kick or short-distance knee or (techniques covered shortly) and finish with a series of counterattacks.

Punch Defense 2

*This technique, similar to punch defense 1, will intercept an incoming
punch while delivering an instantaneous counterstrike over the top of the
incoming punch.*

Stand in your regular-outlet stance. As the punch comes in,
deflect the attacker's arm downward by using an inverted punch
(pinky down, thumb up). You must extend your body reach to its
fullest by pivoting toward your target on the same-side leg as
your deflecting arm. Keep your chin tucked and buried into your
shoulder.

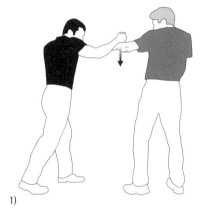

1)

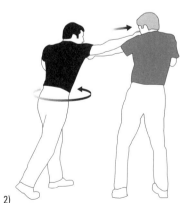

2)

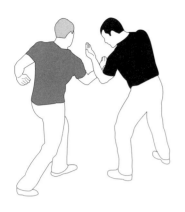

Low Punch Defense

This technique misdirects uppercuts and other low punches

From your left-outlet stance, lower your defending arm to intercept and deflect the uppercut punch that is traveling from low to high. (Note: Another low punch defense, called *gunting,* uses movement 4 of the 360-degree defense to protect your ribs: from your outlet stance, bring your elbows down to form a protective barrier.)

Two-Handed Sliding Block

This technique parries a straight punch to the inside, setting you up to deliver a powerful knee to the groin.

From your left outlet stance, block your attacker's incoming straight punch with your left arm, using the heel of your palm and forearm to push your attacker's incoming right arm to the inside. Follow up with a knee strike to the groin and continue with additional counterattacks.

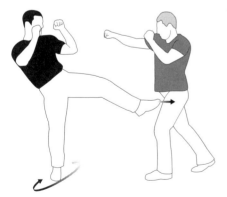

Timing Defenses Against Punches

While challenging to execute, a timing-defensive preemptive strike can also be extremely effective against punch attacks. This technique will preempt your opponent before he can land his punch.

You can execute the technique in one of two ways: either kick or knee your opponent in the knee, groin, or midsection as he tries to punch or strike with straight, roundhouse, or uppercut punches.

Closing and Protecting the Body Against Unexpected Attacks

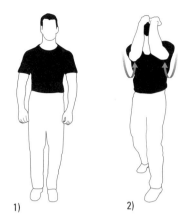

1) 2)

If you are attacked unexpectedly by a hail of incoming blows to your head, your instinctive reaction will be protect yourself by raising your arms to your head. Krav maga *builds on this natural reaction.*

As strikes come in to your head, pull your arms in from your regular-outlet stance to form a defensive shield. Such a cover gives you a moment of protection as you regroup to escape or counterattack. To protect the head, bring both of your arms in front of your face with your forearms out to the side and your palm heels resting on the crown of your skull. The hand positioning is similar to your outlet stance; however, you are trying to seal any openings around your head. (Note: You can also use this "protect and cover" defense when on the ground.) After you regroup, burst forward with an attack of your own.

Perfecting Your Technique

Shadow boxing (known in Hebrew as "*Tzel* (cell) *box*") can enhance your punching skills and fluidity. Practice without any contact. Methods include the following:

1. Use a mirror to practice punch combinations from both a left- and right-outlet stance.
2. Move in and out with combinations using proper footwork.
3. Close your eyes to perform combinations as you envision boxing movements.

Elbow and other Upper Body Strikes

In this section you'll learn numerous strikes with your elbows, along with a few new punches that will teach you the proper body position for a related elbow strike. As you deliver an elbow strike, you may either keep the hand of the striking arm open or clenched in a fist. By keeping the hand open, the muscles are less tense before impact, allowing you to tighten them the split second before impact. A clenched fist tightens the forearm and active muscle groups to increase the strength of impact and help prevent injury but may be slightly slower because of the tensed muscles. Use the hand position that is most comfortable for you prior to delivering the elbow strike. You can achieve the best of both worlds by clenching the fist just prior to impact, while the elbow strike is in motion. This accelerates the strike and conserves energy by not tensing your body longer than necessary.

TRUE KRAVIST

Two female traveling companions were sitting at a bar in Spain. A local suitor put his hands on one of the women's legs. The woman told the man to remove his hands, but instead, he took further liberties. The second female companion, both incensed and trained in *krav maga* jumped from her barstool and delivered a crushing horizontal elbow to the man's neck, knocking him to the floor. She stomped him with her heel for good measure, and then the women made their escape.

The Horizontal Elbow Strike

Similar to the front roundhouse punch, this technique uses the extremely hard surface of the elbow. You will give up reach using the elbow in comparison to the hook punch, but the power and strength behind this upper-body strike is unparalleled.

Execute the front horizontal elbow the same way you would a front roundhouse punch, except, just prior to your explosive pivot, make a fist while bringing the striking hand in toward your clavicle and parallel to the ground. Follow up with a rear horizontal elbow, using the same movement as a rear-hook punch. You can also deliver the horizontal elbow strike from a crouch.

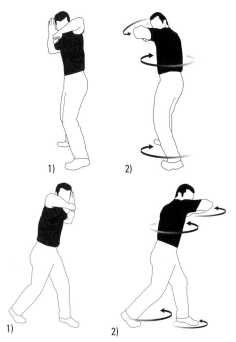

The Lateral Elbow

A lateral elbow strike can attack an opponent who is standing to your side. Use this strike to target the face, jaw, and throat. In addition, depending on height and positioning, you can throw a modified horizontal elbow to the opponent's ribs, midsection, kidneys, and other targets of opportunity.

Practice the technique from either your regular-outlet stance or a passive stance. Position your striking arm similar to the horizontal elbow starting position. Bring your striking arm parallel to the ground while making a fist and draw your forearm close to your body. As with your other combative strikes, synchronize your lower- and upper-body movements. As you deliver the strike, take a short sidestep forward in the same direction your elbow is traveling. This movement shifts the body weight behind the blow. For a right-elbow strike, step to your right; for a left-elbow strike, step to your left. As you step in the direction of your strike, extend the elbow as you make contact. With your rear leg, take the same size step as the forward leg, ending in roughly the same equidistant leg position from which you began. Prior to

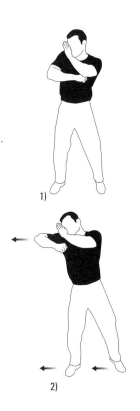

taking the step, bring the hand of your nonstriking elbow in front of your face on the same side as the chambered elbowing arm. This covering movement further protects your face and sets you up for your next combative.

Roundhouse Weapons Strikes

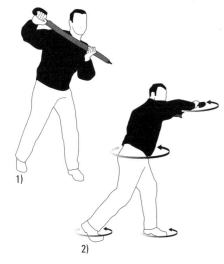

1)

2)

You can use a hook punch or elbow strike movement while wielding a weapon, such as an umbrella, walking stick, chair leg, baton, rifle, or any strong, elongated object you can grip.

Start in a left-outlet stance. Move your lower body and torso in the same explosive rotation as your hook punches and horizontal elbows. Regardless of whether you need one or two hands to wield your weapon, pivot your hip to use the weapon to its full force and effect. For example, if you practice a grip-end (butt) umbrella strike, you cannot hit all the way through to your target without fully pivoting your hips, similar to a baseball or golf swing. Your grip for a two-handed hold should create a large striking surface along the weapon's front tip and end. Your thumbs should face each other so your knuckles are facing upward. (You may also invert the forward hand, which is the preferred grip using a rifle as a blunt, striking weapon.)

Defenses Against Elbow Strikes and Roundhouse Weapons Combatives

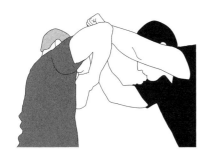

Defending against a front-horizontal elbow and compact-elongated weapons strikes can be challenging.

Block the strike with the fleshy underside of your forearms by rotating the forearms in to meet the strike. The closer you defend to the hand delivering the elbow or holding the weapon, the less impact you will have to absorb.

Weapons of Opportunity 101 ✎

You can use defensive weapons of opportunity and objects of distraction to gain an advantage or level the fighting field. You can distract an opponent simply by spitting into his eye while simultaneously kicking him in the groin. You can also slip off your belt and snap the buckle into at an attacker's eyes or throw liquid into his face while simultaneously delivering a groin kick or other combative.

Displaying a defensive weapon of opportunity, such as brandishing the tip of a long umbrella, might make a would-be aggressor think twice. Consider any weapon an extension of your body, using the same basic motions that you would use during an unarmed confrontation. Keep in mind that your weapon can easily be used against you, so you must learn how to use it properly.

Defensive weapons of opportunity can be loosely grouped into six categories:

1. **Blunt Objects.** Use sticks, flashlights, stones, chairs, magazines, books, garbage can lids, briefcases, bottles, shoes, and wrenches to strike your attacker.
2. **Edged or pointlike objects.** These include broken bottles, keys, scissors, pens, forks, and cooking thermometers, which can all cause serious harm. Use them when he threat requires.
3. **Flexible, elongated objects.** Throw or launch belts, chains, ropes, jackets, and towels against an attacker's face.
4. **Distraction objects and materials.** Throw keys, coins, watches, loose papers, cellular phones, and clothing, toward an attacker's face. You can also spit in the attacker's face to gain a few seconds of distraction, allowing you to run away or follow up with a strike.
5. **Distraction and irritant liquids/sprays.** These include spittle, coffee, perfume, alcohol, and aerosols. Note that certain liquids or sprays may result in a temporary or even permanent blinding effect.
6. **Defensive shield-type objects.** Use chairs, briefcases, duffle bags, garbage lids, and other shieldlike objects to create a barrier between you and your attacker. You can also thrust these toward your attacker and then follow up with a kick.

✎

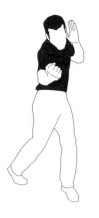

The Uppercut Punch

The uppercut punch can seriously damage your opponent's exposed chin, throat, or groin (when you are on the ground and your opponent is standing).

Stand in the general-outlet stance. Bend your knees slightly to generate power from the lower body, allowing your hips to explode through the target. Pivot the rear leg inward and straighten your knees as you punch, delivering an upward blow from across your body. A common mistake is to drop the arm rather than the body. Deliver the front-uppercut punch the same way, except pivot the front leg inward. Make contact with the first two knuckles, turning your fist toward the opponent so that your palm is facing inward toward you.

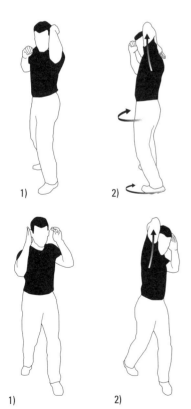

The Uppercut Elbow

Similar to an uppercut punch, this technique uses the forearm to strike upward at the jaw, throat, or chin. You can also use it to attack the groin and abdomen when you are on the ground or lower than your opponent.

Start in a left-outlet stance. Bring the striking arm close to your body and thrust your elbow upward close to your front ear for proper follow-through. You may wish to keep your hand open to avoid striking yourself in the ear.

Reverse Knuckles and Hammer Fist Strikes

These strikes attack an opponent who is standing behind you.

Start in an outlet stance. Turn your head to face your attacker. As you turn to see your attacker, open up your hips in the direction of your strike and begin to spin your body toward your opponent. As your body spins and your hips open up, your striking arm will swing around. Make contact with the first two knuckles, with your pinky facing down. Keep your elbow joint slightly bent to avoid any hyperextension on impact.

A variation of the reverse knuckles punch, the reverse hammer fist, involves using the fleshy part of the closed fist by keeping the knuckles parallel to the ground.

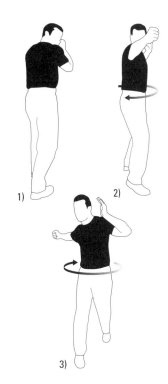

The Horizontal Rear Elbow

The horizontal rear elbow follows the same body movement principles of the reverse knuckles or hammer fist strike.

In this strike your head must lead your body while your hips generate power to deliver this short, compact strike. Bring your elbow into your body with your forearm parallel to the ground. As your turn, either pivot on the balls of your feet or use an open-up step by stepping to the rear with your same-side leg as the arm delivering the elbow to build momentum and power. This rear elbow strike is easily translated into a rear horizontal strike with a blunt weapon such as an umbrella.

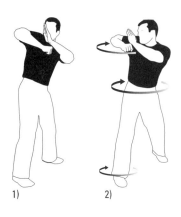

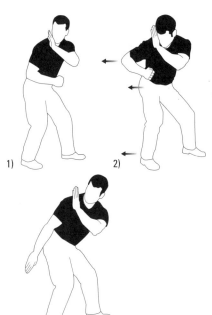

1) 2)

3)

The Perpendicular Rear Elbow

The perpendicular rear elbow delivers a compact strike to an opponent's groin, midsection, face, and other targets. In this strike your hips once again create the power by opening up as you take a short step backward with the leg on the same side.

Start in a regular left-outlet stance. Keeping your striking arm close to your body, look over your shoulder in the direction of your strike. Step back slightly with the same-side leg as your striking arm. As you shift your body weight through the strike, make impact with the elbow to the midsection or groin. You can either keep your hand open or clenched. The perpendicular rear elbow movement is readily applied to using a weapon to thrust behind you.

The Rear Vertical Uppercut Elbow

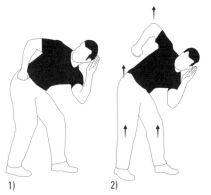

1) 2)

The rear vertical elbow strike is another good follow-up to the short, rear elbow.

Start in the left-outlet stance. With your legs slightly bent, make a fist to strengthen your arms and shoulder. Look where you are striking. Then explode upward with your hips, shoulders, and arm, targeting the solar plexus, throat, and face with the top of your elbow. You can also use a blunt weapon with this strike.

The "Over-the-Top" Elbow

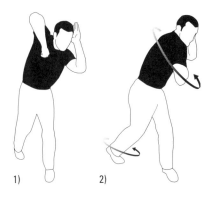

1) 2)

This strike is designed to slam down on your opponent. Targets include the eye ridge, nose, ear, and throat.

The "over-the-top" elbow uses a hip-pivot movement that's somewhere between the one used in the straight punch and roundhouse punch. Beginning from your outlet stance, bring the striking elbow up and over, rotating "over the top" or from high to low. This strike is especially effective when you are able to trap an opponent's forward arm with your forward arm. You can then clamp down the opponent's defense to attack vulnerable target areas. You can also use a weapon to strike "over the top"; however, your arms should not cross but, instead, move in a parallel motion.

The Downward Hammer Fist

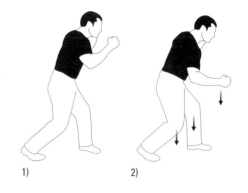

The downward hammer fist usually targets the back of the neck but can also be used against the face, groin, kidneys, and in-between the shoulder blades, depending on the opponent's position.

From your left-outlet stance, drop your body weight by bending your knees and simultaneously bring your fist down on your target, moving your body in concert. Do not bring your arm higher than you would position it in your regular-outlet stance. A weapon can be brought down on a target in the same way.

The Downward Elbow Strike

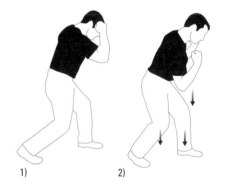

This strike is similar to the vertical hammer fist. Targets again include the back of the neck, in-between the shoulder blades and kidneys. If your opponent is on the ground, his face and groin can become targets.

From your left-outlet stance, execute the same motion as a vertical hammer fist, but this time connect with your elbow. Do not bring your arm higher than you would position it in your regular-outlet stance.

Attacking Sensitive Areas

In addition to punching and elbowing your opponent, you can also use your fingers, thumbs, and many other parts of your upper body to inflict a great amount of damage, especially if you target vulnerable areas such as the eyes, groin, throat, and fingers. Although simple to learn and execute, the techniques in this section will become a valuable part of your *krav maga* arsenal.

Groin Strike with the Hand

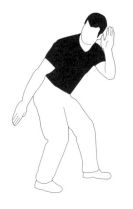

A highly effective follow-up strike to the perpendicular rear elbow, or an independent strike in its own right, this striketargets one of the body's most sensitive areas.

To strike the groin with your hand, cup your hand. You may strike forward, to the side, or to the rear by keeping the fingertips down toward the ground. By whipping your hand into the groin, you create a potent, debilitating blow. You can also use a hammer fist by clenching the fingers into a fist for more power. You can also attack an opponent's groin when facing him in the same way by cupping your hand and striking with the palm out.

Eye Gouges

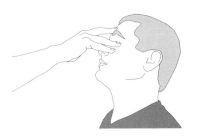

Finger strikes to the eyes can disable an opponent quickly and effectively. The eyeball can be collapsed with minimum pressure. Blinding or partially blinding an attacker sets up retzev *follow-up strikes to end a confrontation quickly.*

For a multiple-finger strike, fold your fingers slightly inward toward your palm and spread them just enough so they do not touch. This will reduce the possibility of injuring them on impact. If the impact is hard, flexing the fingers inward will collapse them into their natural articulation. Note that the fingers are fragile and can easily be fractured even when taking precautions. Execute the strike with a body movement similar to your straight punches, with the fingers making contact with the eyes.

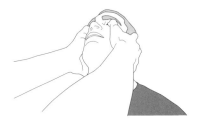

You can also strike the eyes with your thumbs, penetrating the eye socket. Use your opponent's cheekbone as a guide. A rule

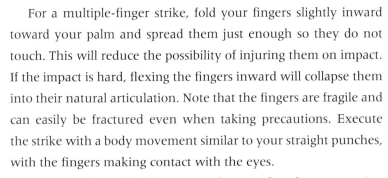

of thumb (pardon the pun): if you can find the cheekbone, you can find the eye. This is particularly important if you are not in a position to see your attacker, such as a ground-fighting situation or if it is dark. You can insert one or both of your thumbs into your opponent's eye sockets.

The Educational Defense

This technique tells a would-be assailant that you are trained; hence, its name "educational defense." The educational defense attacks the hollow of your opponent's neck, one of the most vulnerable areas of the body when it can be reached.

Elongate the forward arm to apply finger pressure with a slight bend in the fingers to the hollow of the attacker's neck. While elongating the arm, take a step back with opposite leg, keeping the majority of your weight on the forward leg and your chin tucked. Pivot on the same-side leg of the arm, thrusting your hip and shoulder forward to meet the threat. For this defense, you will not have time to step toward your target, but, instead, will have to step back. Keep your weight over your forward leg. You can also use weapons of opportunity such as a pen or cell phone against the hollow of the neck (and other parts of the neck).

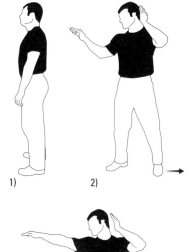

1) 2) 3)

Whipping Blows

A finger eye-whip strike attacks your opponent's eyes with your finger-tips. This technique requires great care to avoid injuring the fingertips against the forehead or other facial bones.

As you strike, keep your fingers and wrist flexible. An over-hand whip keeps the striking hand's thumb pointing up and pinky facing down. Make contact with the tips of the index and middle fingers. Whipping motions can also be used against an opponent's exposed neck to stun him for follow-up *retzev* counterattacks.

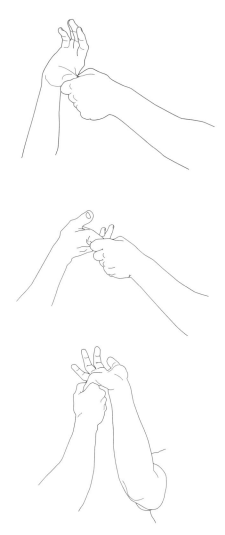

Finger Manipulations and Breaks

Finger manipulations and breaks are easy to learn. As with all joints, the fingers follow a natural articulation. When forced out of their natural articulation, great discomfort ensues. Enough force will disable a finger's movement by dislocating or breaking it.

A thumb grab is an effective way to control an opponent. One of the best ways to understand these conclusions is to gently manipulate your own set of fingers with your opposite hand. Once you grab a finger, extend it back toward the elbow. You will quickly understand the finger's natural movements.

To achieve the best result in finger manipulations and breaks, the finger joint(s) must be isolated. You will notice that you have a much greater degree of flexibility in your fingers if you hold your "experimental hand" below the wrist. The wrist allows for more flexibility in the fingers. By holding or isolating the hand above the wrist, you will notice a much more limited degree of flexibility while the pain will set in more quickly.

TRUE KRAVIST

A young man trained in *krav maga* sensed a youth was trying to reach into his pocket to steal his wallet. Rather than striking the youth, the man grabbed the youth's finger and bent it enough to create discomfort. This simple move dissuaded the rest of the pickpocket's friends from tangling with the *krav maga* practitioner.

Combination Workout Drill

The following drill will help you to learn most of the upper-body techniques in combination. After a short warmup, practice each combination twenty times from both the left- and right-outlet stances. Then cool down with some stretching.

1. Straight front/rear arm-punch combinations.
2. Thrusting lead-arm finger strike (to jolt the head back to expose the neck) followed by a rear punch to the exposed throat.
3. Straight front/rear, arm-punch combinations followed by left front/rear, arm-roundhouse-punch combinations.
4. Straight front/rear arm-punch combinations, followed by front/rear, arm-roundhouse-punch combinations, followed by left/right (front/rear), uppercut-punch combinations.
5. Low/high roundhouse punch with same arm and opposite arm combinations.
6. Straight punch and roundhouse punch or horizontal-elbow combination with the same arm.
7. Roundhouse punch with forward arm and straight punch with the rear arm.
8. Roundhouse punch with forward arm and uppercut with rear arm.
9. Straight punch with forward arm and uppercut with same arm.
10. Uppercut with forward arm and roundhouse with same arm.
11. Horizontal elbow followed by the opposite arm's horizontal elbow.
12. Horizontal elbow followed by the opposite arm's horizontal elbow.
13. Forward arm vertical elbow followed by the rear arm's horizontal elbow.
14. Forward horizontal elbow followed by the rear arm's vertical elbow.
15. Straight multiple-finger eye gouges followed by horizontal elbows.
16. Side elbow followed by the opposite arm's horizontal elbow.
17. Any combination of these.

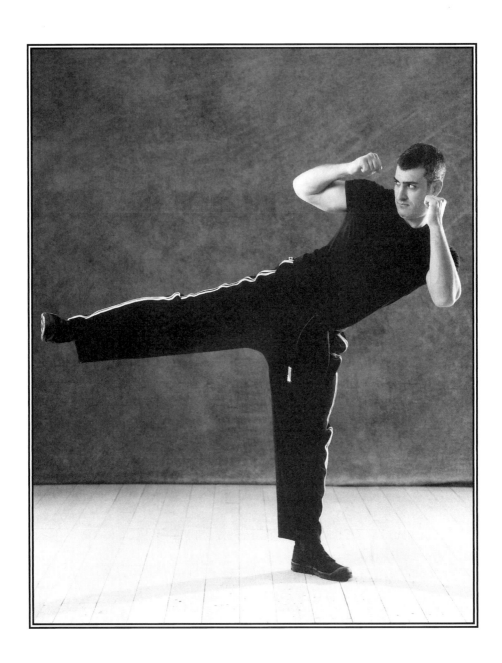

CHAPTER 5

Mastering Lower-Body Strikes and Kicks

Use your body's most powerful muscles to send your attacker packing

Your lower body houses the most powerful fighting weapons that you can use while at your maximum fighting range. Your knees and the balls of your feet (especially when clad in shoes) serve as hard and durable striking surfaces. When you kick or knee your opponent, you use your body's largest muscle groups, including the gluteus, quadriceps, and hamstrings. If, as with punching, you put your entire body mass and strength behind your kick or knee, you can deliver a devastating blow, no matter your size or weight.

You can perform *krav maga* kicks at low, mid-body, and head-level heights. To execute high kicks, you'll need a lot of flexibility, as well as enough strength in your outer thighs to lift your leg. If you lack the flexibility and strength to kick high, don't fret. In developing its self-defense, close-quarters-combat program, the IDF forced test candidates to run extensive distances with full combat loads. Many of these test candidates were accomplished martial artists who favored high kicks to the head. After an exhausting run in combat gear, the candidates were told to defend against an attack using whatever techniques they felt most comfortable. Few of the candidates skilled in high kicks could perform them. Their physical taxation prior to the fighting tests made it extremely difficult to kick high. The IDF recognized the need to use only self-defense, close-quarters-combat techniques that would work for all trainees, especially under trying circumstances. Therefore, low kicks combined with upper-body combatives be-

FIGHTING FIT

Shari Winnick, a *krav maga* student for the past three years, offers this account of what she's gained from practicing *krav maga*:

After just a few weeks of hitting pads, and doing *retzev* in the air, the change in my body was apparent. Not only did my weekly *krav maga* workouts define my muscles, but my overall posture and body composition exuded strength and confidence.

This experience is like nothing I've ever had at the gym before. Cardio-kickboxing classes always made me break a sweat, but they never corrected or even stressed technique at all. In contrast, *krav maga* focuses on mastering proper technique while simultaneously burning calories through constant motion and repetition. In terms of getting a great workout (and also defending myself in a bad situation), this is far more important.

The *krav maga* curriculum has also enhanced my other fitness activities, including running and core strengthening. Throughout my three years of training, *krav maga* has given me many physical and mental rewards: better muscle definition, endurance, alertness, and self-confidence.

came integral to *krav maga* training. These are difficult to defend against.

For straight kicks you'll make contact with the ball of your foot. To accustom your feet to striking, curl your toes up toward you and repeatedly tap the ground with the ball of your foot. Increase the force of your taps, turning them into modified kicks, as you become more comfortable with this foot positioning. To strike with your heel for a stomp, arch your toes toward your knee to expose the heel. Perform the same tapping exercise to accustom your heel to striking. Note that this heel exercise is a combative kick in itself, the stomp, useful when an opponent is on the ground and you are standing.

For all straight kicks and knees think of your kneecap as a directional finder or pointer. Wherever the knee is pointed, the kick or knee will follow. Hip alignment is paramount to keeping your leg on target. Note: Do not fully extend the kicking leg unless you are impacting a target. Rather, extend only about 90 percent. As with punches, you risk hyperextending your knee by locking the joint. For all kicks and knees, shift your body weight toward your target. This will maximize your impact.

The Rear Straight Offensive Kick

Kicking with your rear leg will connect with enormous power to your opponent's knee, groin, abdomen, and midsection. Higher targets include the solar plexus, the neck, and the head.

To practice the basic rear kick movement, from your left-outlet stance, take the longest possible step forward with your right leg. As you step, turn out your left foot approximately 90 degrees. Notice how your body elongates and your nonkicking base leg naturally pivots out, with your toes pointed to your left. (Although the optimal turn is 90 degrees, some people experience knee discomfort when they turn the knee this far.) Turning out your front leg will thrust the hips of your rear, base leg

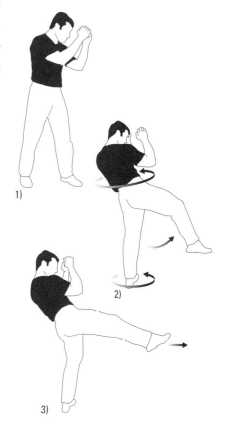

1)

2)

3)

forward, giving you maximum extension and power using *glicha*: "a sliding step" with your rear leg that carries your body weight through the kick. This enables you to throw your body mass behind the kick.

Launch the kick from low to high or "under the radar screen" of your opponent's vision. Connect with the ball of your foot against your target. Do not raise the knee up and then push out to kick. Rather, snap or thrust the kick toward the target. Land, after impact, with your kicking leg forward. Keep your hands up the entire time. Many people unconsciously drop their hands to improve their balance. (Note: You can practice keeping your hands up by grabbing your shirt collar as you kick).

Front Straight Offensive Kick

For this front kick you'll use kicking and basic leg movements similar to those used for the rear kick to maximize your reach and kicking power.

Kicking with your front leg can connect with great power to your opponent's knee, groin, abdomen, and midsection. Higher targets include the solar plexus, neck, and the head.

As you did for your rear offensive kick, from your left-outlet stance, take a maximum step with your left leg and remain in that position. You will notice how your body elongates again and your nonkicking base leg pivots in approximately a 90-degree angle with your toes pointed to your right. Whip your front leg out as though you are thrusting the ball of your foot through a target, again "under the radar screen." As you kick, keep your hands up to protect your head. To enhance your footwork and balance, learn to deliver the kick and then recover into your left-outlet stance. In addition, as your kicking leg touches the ground, you may also use the retreating footwork you learned with your straight punches to move your body backward.

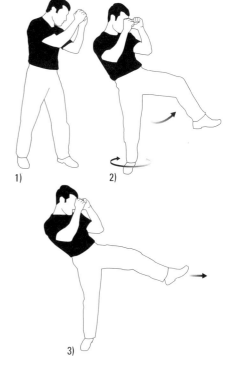

Shuffle Front-Leg Straight Kick

A "shuffle" front-leg straight kick is highly effective if you require a longer range strike.

Start in a left-outlet stance. Kick with your front foot while simultaneously shuffling forward with your rear foot to same spot your front foot had just occupied. In other words, your rear foot replaces your foot by moving to the spot where your front foot was previously. As a result your entire body weight shifts forward—as with all kicks—while your body moves through the kick. Practice this shuffle of the feet, or *secoul,* while moving both forward and backward.

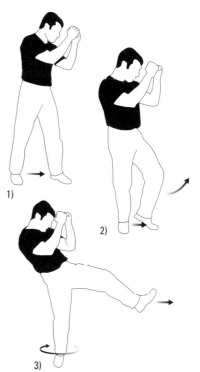

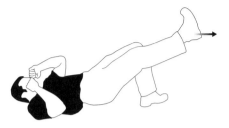

Straight Kicks When on the Ground

Even when you're on the ground, you can successfully launch a modified front-straight kick against an opponent who is standing.

As soon as you fall to the ground, protect your head, using arm positioning similar to your outlet stance to form your defensive posture. Although you may periodically drop your arms to the ground to move your body back away from your opponent or rotate your body to meet a threat from a different angle, keep your arms in a protective position for your head as often as you can. As you kick, keep your base leg against the ground for lever-

---

Lower-Body Drills

To familiarize yourself with lower-body techniques, practice the following drill. Use the straight kick or substitute any lower-body technique you wish to learn.

1. From the left-outlet stance: 20 kicks with the forward left leg and 20 kicks with the rear right leg pivoting correctly on the base leg while simultaneously placing your hands in the correct fighting position.
2. From the right-outlet stance: 20 kicks with the forward right leg and 20 kicks with the rear left leg, pivoting correctly on your base leg while simultaneously placing your hands in the correct fighting position.
3. From the left-outlet stance: 20 right/left switching-kick combinations, pivoting correctly on the respective base legs while simultaneously placing your hands in the correct fighting position.
4. From the right-outlet stance: 20 kicks left/right switching kick combinations, pivoting correctly on the respective base legs while simultaneously placing your hands in the correct fighting position.

age. Thrust out the kick with your other leg. Use your upper back and shoulders as a launching platform, putting your entire torso behind the kick and allowing your torso to lift off the ground. Make contact with either the heel or ball of your foot and recoil quickly to avoid having your leg caught by your opponent. Launching this kick from the ground becomes an offensive movement, due to your angle of attack against a standing opponent.

The Front and Rear Straight Knee

Once you know how to kick, you know how to knee. Knee attacks provide some of the most punishing strikes and a strong finish to any technique.

You will knee your opponent with the same technique you use to kick. Rather than make contact with your foot, however, you will ram your kneecap into your target. Rechambering your knee, by returning to your outlet stance, allows for additional powerful and debilitating strikes. (Note: for advanced weapons-defense techniques, after the initial disarm, knees may not be appropriate as they may collide with a blade or cross in front of a firearm.)

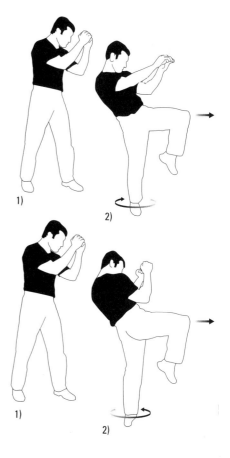

1)

2)

1)

2)

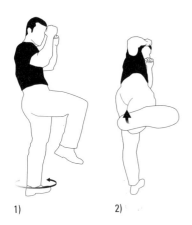

1)   2)

The Side Kick

The side kick and rear defensive kick build your arsenal of combatives, enabling you to kick a threat to your side or rear. The side kick and rear defensive kicks will become some of your most formidable striking weapons. The side kick is highly effective against lateral attacks, such as straight punches, where you can use the kick's superior reach and power against the attacker's forward knee, thighs, or midsection.

By varying your outlet stance or "cheating" by positioning your feet almost perpendicular to your opponent, the side kick can target an opponent in front of you. Execute the side kick with your front leg, which is closer to your target. Once again, pivoting and aligning the base leg in the appropriate direction is essential to maximize reach and power.

Defending Against Straight Kicks 101

When learning any kind of defense, think of your own offensive capabilities and how you would defend against them. Advanced *krav maga* training prepares you to overcome a defense to your offense creating a special kind of fighting "chess game." Your regular-outlet stance allows you to defend against a myriad attacks without compromising your ability to defend other parts of your body should they be attacked simultaneously.

Imagine your response if someone were to kick at your groin. You'd probably drop your hands and contort your body, bringing one leg across the other to protect your groin. *Krav maga* builds on this response, but modifies your action. For this particular defense, do not drop your hands because this will leave your face open to attack. In the following pages, you'll learn how to use your natural instincts to defend against groin kicks and other incoming attacks.

To execute the kick, raise your front kicking leg until your leg is bent 90 degrees and your thigh is parallel to the ground. Deliver the kick by thrusting your raised leg out, pointing the heel toward the target and curling the toes toward your body. Keep your foot parallel with the ground as you make contact. As with every other kick, your body weight must shift forward into your target.

Note: You can cover ground and set up the proper distance for the kick by stepping your rear foot toward your target just before you launch the kick. This is called a "stepping side kick," or *secoul* in Hebrew.

Side Kick While on the Ground

The side kick works well if you find yourself on the ground on your side with your attacker standing over you. The attacker's knees, thighs, and groin usually present the best targets when in this position.

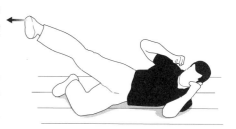

Keep both hands raised in a defensive posture and one leg on the ground. Kick sideways on an upward motion, curling your toes toward you and connecting with your heel. You may wish to place one forearm on the ground to establish a strong kicking base with good balance. Keep your nonkicking leg flush against the ground prior to the kick. As you kick, this base leg may rise slightly off the ground to give you leverage.

Note: you can also use a side kick-like motion or the "brakes" to defend against a mount. Pull your top knee into your torso so that your foreleg and shin can act as "brakes" against an attacker trying to get on top of you. By extending out, you create separation and may be able to push your attacker away.

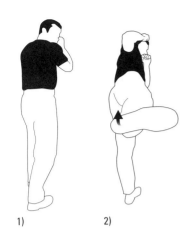

1)　　　　2)

Rear Defensive Kick

Targets for rear defensive kicks include the knees, thighs, groin, midsection, and solar plexus. Higher kicks can target the neck and head.

To recognize a threat from behind, turn your head in the direction of your attacker. Even though your upper torso will naturally lean away from the kick, you must drive your body through the kick. Thrust your foot into your target, connecting with your heel, as you did with the side kick. You may connect with your foot parallel to the ground or with your toes pointed to the ground.

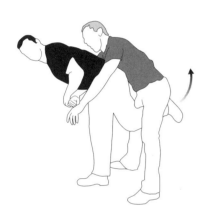

Mule Kick

Another highly effective kick, the mule kick, uses an upward kicking motion with your heel to connect with your opponent's groin when he is standing behind you in close proximity.

From your regular left-outlet stance, shift your body weight over one leg. Quickly bend the knee of your free leg, as if you were going to kick yourself in the buttock. Deliver the strike with an upward arching motion and hit the most opportune target, including the shin, groin, abdomen, or head.

Rear Roundhouse Kick

This swift and powerful combative strike targets the opponent's vulnerable leg areas. The medium-height roundhouse kick targets the groin, midsection, ribs, and kidneys, whereas a high roundhouse kick targets the neck and head.

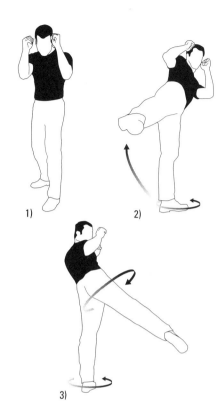

From your left-outlet stance, raise your right rear leg and then rotate the knee, thigh, and shin parallel to the ground. Pivot on the ball of your left base leg foot so that your body turns to the right, in the direction of your pivoting kneecap. If your pivot is correct, you will end up with your buttocks facing an imaginary opponent in front of you. You must swivel your head to keep your eyes on your target. Continue to pivot and swing around toward your opponent as you straighten and strengthen your kicking leg to simulate the kick. As with your other combative strikes, your entire weight comes through the kick as your body torques through the target. As your body turns, keep your eyes on your target. As you kick, your hip must "roll over" or rotate parallel to the ground so that your foot is nearly parallel to the ground.

You can connect with either your shin or with the ball of your foot. If you use your shin, which is my preferred method because it provides a hard, durable striking surface, extend your toes and straighten your leg and attack the Achilles tendon, knee joint, thigh, or midsection. If you kick with the ball of your foot, pull back the toes and keep your foot parallel to the ground. Although the foot is more fragile than the shin, this second option provides a more precise striking surface, ideal for striking the groin.

To facilitate the kick and accelerate the pivot, you can also take a step out with the base leg to set up the roundhouse kick rather than spinning on the ball of your foot. This shortcut is particularly useful for low, powerful sweeps against an attacker's Achilles tendon.

Note: You can easily convert a roundhouse shin kick into a sweep by lowering your center of gravity to target the opponent's Achilles tendon just above the ankle.

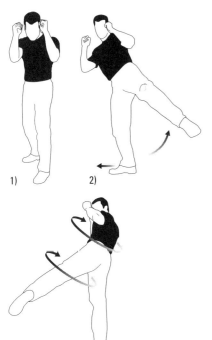

Front Roundhouse Kick

Similar to the rear roundhouse, you'll execute this kick with your front leg. The front roundhouse kick is a particularly effective quick kick because of your proximity to your opponent.

You'll execute this kick in the same manner as the rear roundhouse kick using a step with your base leg, except your rear leg now becomes your base leg. As with the rear roundhouse kick, your body must swing through the kick to maximize its impact.

Roundhouse Knee

Similar to a roundhouse kick, the knee best targets the kidneys and ribs.

You will use the same technique and movement for the front and rear roundhouse knees as you do for the front and rear roundhouse kicks, except you will not extend your leg, and you will connect with your kneecap instead of your shin or foot. Always keep your hands up as you move.

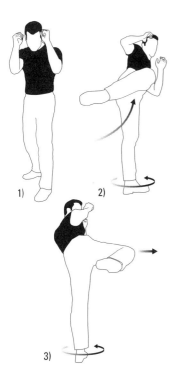

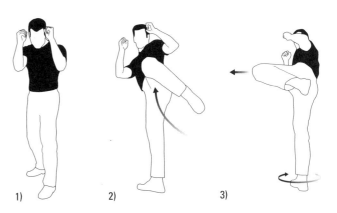

The Shin Deflection

This move redirects a low, straight kick.

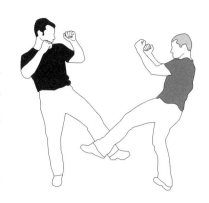

From your regular-outlet stance, use your foreleg to deflect or parry an incoming kick without dropping your hands. Slide your front leg across your body while maintaining your balance, but do not overcommit your front leg, which may throw you off balance and, more important, put you in a vulnerable position. Once you successfully parry the kick, remain in your outlet stance and prepare for a *retzev* counter attack.

The Intercepting Side Kick

This defense against a low straight kick requires specific timing to intercept the kick with your front foot.

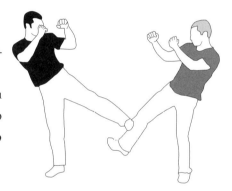

From your regular-outlet stance, raise your front leg and turn your foot parallel to the ground, using your foot's entire length to intercept your opponent's kicking foot before it has a chance to fully launch.

The Inside Knee/Shin Bar

Similar to the technique used in a side kick on the ground, the knee/shin bar defends against a knee attack by blocking or braking your opponent's incoming knee. Defenses against knee attacks require a great amount of timing.

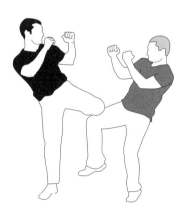

From your regular-outlet stance, rotate your forward or brace your leg 90 degrees until your shin is perpendicular to your opponent's thigh. Push it into the thigh as you trap your opponent's knee. Keep your body weight forward and your bracing leg parallel to your opponent's torso as you lean into him. Follow up with simultaneous *retzev* upper-body counterattacks.

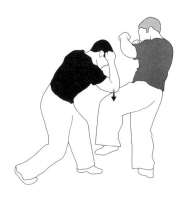

Gunting

This technique uses an elbow strike to defend against an incoming knee strike.

From your regular outlet stance, apply a modified vertical-downward elbow block and intercept the incoming knee with the tip of your elbow. If properly executed, the elbow will strike the opponent's quadriceps, causing significant pain.

Roundhouse Kick Defenses

Before you can defend against a low roundhouse kick, you must see it coming. As with low-straight-kick defenses, you will always defend with your forward leg regardless if your opponent kicks with his front or rear leg.

Krav maga does not use shin-against-shin blocks and shin-against-shin attacks for roundhouse kicks. Direct shin-to-shin contact is not suitable for most trainees who have not spent time toughening their shins. (Recall that the shin defense against the low, straight kick is a deflection and not a direct-impact defense where the shin must absorb the strike's impact, similar to redirecting the straight punch.)

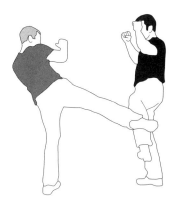

Low-Roundhouse-Kick Defense

In this defense you'll use your shin to meet your opponent's roundhouse kick at his foot.

To execute the defense, open your front hip wide enough to the outside to parry your opponent's foot with your shin. You must have a strong-enough base and good balance to defend against this kick. As the kick comes in, block it with your shin.

After blocking the kick, immediately execute counterattacks, such as a knee to the attacker's exposed groin.

Medium Roundhouse Defense

When possible you can catch your opponent's kicking leg, which will place your opponent in a highly vulnerable position for your retzev counterattacks. He is now forced to balance on one leg while you have his other leg secured tightly underneath your armpit.

From your outlet stance, take a 30-degree rear–side step as you move the arm closest to your attacker down to catch your opponent's leg. This side step moves you to the end of the kick's follow-through, allowing you to absorb only about one-third of the kick's power in the midsection. To execute the step correctly, exhale as you step away from the kick. Do not drag your near leg, but step out by positioning on the ball of your foot with your knee facing your opponent.

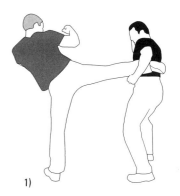
1)

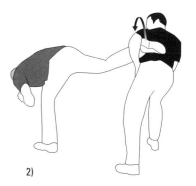
2)

What to Do If Your Opponent 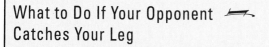 Catches Your Leg

If your opponent catches *your* leg, immediately close the distance to your opponent by bending the knee of your caught leg. Counterattack as soon as possible with eye gouges, strikes, or a jumping clinch by grabbing the opponent's head to position your body to defend a takedown.

An advanced variation involves catching the opponent's leg with a glancing deflection using the heel of your palm. You must execute this technique carefully to prevent breaking your hand.

Immediately execute counterattacks using groin strikes, strikes, or a takedown (discussed in more detail later) by stepping behind the opponent's base leg and forcing him backward.

High-Roundhouse-Kick Defense

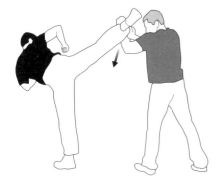

This technique defends against a roundhouse kick to the head.

As the kick comes in toward your head, bury your chin in your shoulder and modify your arm position. Meet the attack with your outside forearm while moving in toward your opponent to deliver a punch to the face, followed by *retzev* counterattacks. Bursting inside in this manner moves you away from the kick's most dangerous angle, where its power is greatest, at the end of the leg. As you move in, keep your forearm angled toward you to encourage the kick to slide up the forearm rather than come directly at the forearm.

Timing Defenses

You can use this defense to sweep the attacker's groin or base leg as the kick comes in.

If you recognize the roundhouse kick early enough, execute a preemptory straight kick with your front leg to the groin or roundhouse kick to the attacker's base leg.

Kick, Knee, and Punching Drills

With the upper- and lower-body combative strikes now part of your arsenal, you now have a number of attack combinations at your disposal. Execute them seamlessly and opportunely when a target or opening becomes available. When combining a kick with an upper-body strike, timing becomes important. After your kick has landed, but before your kicking leg hits the ground, you should already be moving into your next combative. This coordinated movement allows you to capitalize on your first strike's momentum.

Complete 20 repetitions of each of the following drills:

1. Straight front kick forward with *glicha* (a "shuffle step"), punch with same-side arm, straight punch from the rear arm, rear knee.
2. Straight rear kick with forward (into opposite-outlet stance), punch with same-side and rear arm, knee with rear leg.
3. Front roundhouse kick, front straight punch, rear straight punch, rear-roundhouse kick.
4. Side kick with the front leg and reverse-knuckles punch.

Put these strikes together in various other combinations in a continuous flow to form the basis for *retzev* counterattacks.

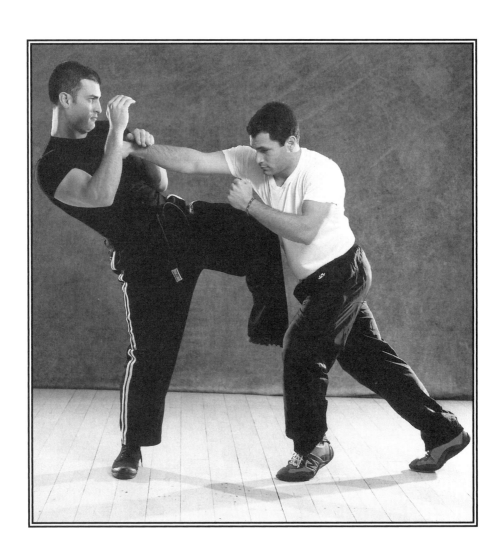

CHAPTER 6

Mastering Close-Contact Fighting

Learn the art of falling, retreating, clinching, throwing, and more

In this chapter you will learn one of the most important techniques of all—how to fall to the ground safely. At some point during a confrontation, you may get your legs knocked out from under you, lose your balance, or trip while running. No matter what causes the fall, you need to know how to go from upright to prone without hurting yourself. Just as important, the techniques you will soon learn will also help you break any type of fall, whether you slip on ice or trip over a curb.

In addition to learning the safest way to fall, you'll also discover how to defend against the most common types of close-contact street attacks, such as throws, grabs, and clinches. You'll also learn how to take down an attacker.

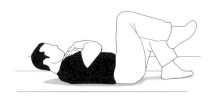

1)

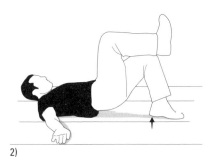

2)

Backward Fall Break

By using your body to create the broadest possible striking surface against the ground, the backward fall break will reduce your impact with the ground, distributing the force of the fall through the more durable areas of your body: the gluteus, lateral muscles, and your forearms. The importance of this safety technique reaches well beyond self-defense applications. For example, the next time you slip on a sheet of ice, the backward fall break will come in handy.

Lie flat on your back. Initially you may prefer to do this on carpeting. You can also use a bed. As you progress in the technique's training steps, however, the bed will bounce you back up, interfering with the learning process. Tuck your chin into your chest so that the back of your head rises off the ground. Cross your arms to form a forty-five-degree angle with one arm overlapping the other on your chest.

Now you're ready to simulate the impact of a fall. Quickly extend your arms out to your sides, 45 degrees below chest level, with your palms down and fingers together. Slap the ground with your arms as you exhale from your lower abdomen. Exhaling on impact creates a vacuum that prevents having the wind knocked out during the fall. Raise one leg as though you were going to deliver a straight defensive kick from the ground. This will protect your tailbone and spine from impact. Prop yourself on the ball of the other foot with your heel off the ground to gain your balance. This is the position into which you want to fall to protect your head, spine, and tailbone from serious injury.

Practice tucking your chin, slapping the ground, exhaling, and raising one leg several times from your crossed arms position on your back. Once you can coordinate the movements, practice from a low squat, letting yourself fall backward. Once you can coordinate your movements from a squatting position, practice from differing heights and eventually from standing.

Side Fall Break

The side fall break prepares you in case you must fall to your side.

For the side fall break, you must slap the ground with the arm closest to the ground, using the same slapping motion as in the rear fall break. As you fall, elevate the same-side leg to avoid having your knee crash to the ground. Stay on the ball of the foot of your other leg and exhale on impact. Practice this fall break in the same manner you did your rear fall break: first, from a lying position; then a squatting position; and finally, a standing position.

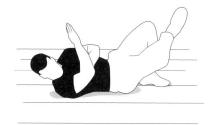

1)

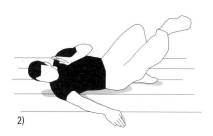

2)

Forward "Soft" Fall Break

The forward "soft" fall break gently brings you to the ground when you are falling forward.

Start in a modified push-up position with your fingers facing inward. Turn your head to one side to prevent your face from hitting the ground. Once secure in this position you can dip a knee to help you rise to your feet quickly or roll over on your back into a defensive fighting posture, if necessary. Initially, you can practice this technique against a wall to familiarize this movement, pushing away from the wall and landing in this modified push-up position. Once you feel comfortable, you can do this movement from a kneeling position and eventually from a standing position.

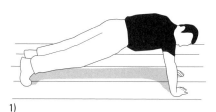

1)

Note: If you've fallen to the ground to duck away from gunfire or an explosion, cover your head with your arms and cross your ankles tightly to protect your groin. Also, try to flatten yourself as much as possible.

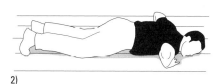

2)

The Body-"Snaking" Retreat

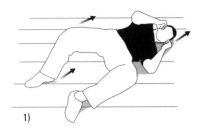

1)

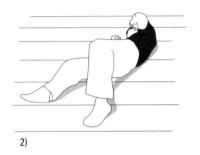

2)

From your defensive posture as practiced with straight kicks from the ground, you can create separation from your opponent by snaking your body (sliding backward), all the while maintaining a strong defensive position.

Lie on your back. Raise your right shoulder blade, and push yourself backward with the ball of your right foot. Protect your head by positioning your arms as you would in a standing-outlet stance. Keep your left foot flush against the ground, and be prepared to dig your heel into the ground for traction. Repeat the process with your left shoulder blade and left foot. Inch back, switching from side to side. Once you get used to snaking, practice the technique while delivering alternating side kicks to protect and separate yourself from your opponent.

Rear-Crawling Retreat

The rear-crawling retreat offers yet another escape option when you find yourself on your back.

Lie on your back. Partially sit up and dig your heels and the heels of your palms into the ground, pushing yourself back with all four limbs and dragging your buttocks with you. In essence, you are scampering backward.

Clinching

A fight can often begin from a clinch, when both opponents are still standing and locked up. The clinch can be advantageous to one opponent and disastrous for another opponent, depending on positioning and respective skill sets.

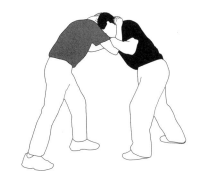

From a regular-outlet stance, position your hands on the crown of your opponent's head inside both of his arms. Do not interlock your fingers. Control your opponent by exerting pressure on the back of the head, near the crown, pulling your opponent toward you. The clinch places you in a strong position to strike your opponent with your knees and then transition to elbow strikes. In addition, it allows you to position your opponent for a throw or takedown.

Takedowns

Krav maga teaches simple and effective takedowns that usually flow from other techniques to put an opponent on the ground. Think of these techniques as extensions of a previously completed combative technique, such as a gouge to the eyes to disorient your opponent as you perform an outside reverse sweep as described below. Although more advanced hip throws and other takedowns are an integral part of advanced *krav maga* training, they are beyond the scope of this book. Practice your takedowns with a partner in a large, open space. Make sure you have enough room to fall without hitting your head on furniture. Use a padded mat to cushion your fall.

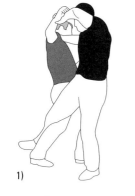

1)

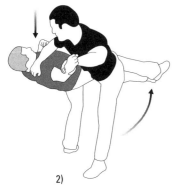

2)

Outside Reverse Sweep

For this technique you'll take out an opponent's legs by sweeping your outside leg against and into the opponent's inside knees or lower legs. You'll combine the sweep with a strike, shove, or hook to the neck. You can target one or both of the opponent's legs and knees.

Stand with your right side to your opponent's left side. Straighten and strengthen your right leg to sweep your opponent's right leg. Grab your opponent's left wrist with your left hand and place your right hand on his shoulder. Push your opponent forward with your hands as you bring your heel back and up against the bend of his knee or Achilles tendon in a chopping motion. Jolt your opponent forward while simultaneously sweeping back. This technique will take your opponent's upper body forward and his lower body back. You must time this move exquisitely well to sweep your opponent before he can counter the move and sweep you first. After your opponent goes down, follow up with kicks and stomps to the head, neck, solar plexus, ribs, groin, fingers, and other targets of opportunity.

Note: You can also hook your same-side arm around your opponent and use it to pull him in toward you as you sweep backward through his nearside leg.

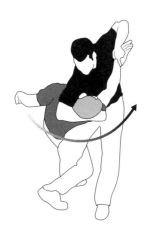

Leg-Hook Takedown w/Same-Side Leg

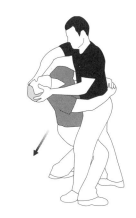

In this takedown you will hook your outside leg to your opponent's outside leg and drive him backward at a 45-degree angle. Because the body is accustomed to moving straight, to the right and left, and to a lesser extent backward, the body's sense of balance is disrupted when forced unexpectedly in an "off-angle" direction, especially backward and to the side.

Stand with your left side to your opponent's right side. Wrap your left leg around the outside of your opponent's right leg. Place the ball of your foot on the ground and strengthen your leg. Then jolt him backward by gouging him in the eyes or pushing upward on his nose, jolting him back on a 45-degree angle in the direction of your hooked foot. Once your opponent is on the ground, move to his dead side as quickly as possible and follow up with additional strikes.

Defenses Against a Tackle

The tackle type of takedown, designed to put an opponent on his back and the attacker in a strong position to continue an attack, is a common takedown used by trained and untrained fighters, especially ground fighters. A tackle takedown can smash you into a wall or put you on the ground quickly with your attacker on top of you. If taken down, your foremost concern must be to protect your head by tucking your chin and doing your best to execute the rear fall break.

To defend against the tackle, you should know how a proper tackle takedown is made. As with other combatives, the tackle's power comes from his hips and legs exploding into the target. Run toward the opponent with your knees bent and body crouched low. Drive your shoulder into your opponent's hips or midsection, with your head to one side of the opponent's torso. Optimally, wrap your arms around the opponent's legs at the

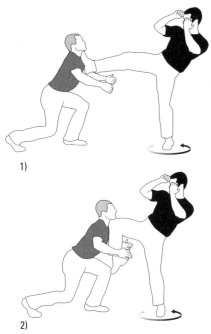

1)

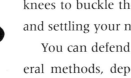

2)

knees to buckle them. Bull your neck by raising your shoulders and settling your neck into them while keeping your face up.

You can defend yourself against a takedown tackle using several methods, depending on how soon you recognize the impending threat. They include the following:

Straight Offensive Kick or Knee-to-the-Face: If you recognize a tackle takedown attack early enough, launch a straight kick or knee (preferably a rear) to the attacker's groin or face. Note that accomplished ground fighters train to overcome this technique by deflecting the kick and continuing with the tackle or takedown.

Side Step Body Defense with Combatives: If you do not have time or are caught unprepared, use a body-defense movement as you control the attacker's head, which will break the angle of attack. For practice purposes, use a sideways body defense to the left by pivoting your right leg 180 degrees. Extend both arms, touching your hands together and cupping your hands outward to give you a strong brace against the attacker's incoming head. Jam the heels of your hands into the side of the attacker's head as you step sideways to break the angle of attack. Follow up with additional strikes. Even if the attacker has long arms and wraps an arm around you, your outstretched arms should provide a strong enough base to control his head.

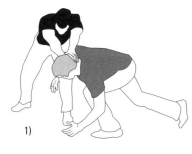

1)

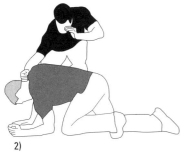

2)

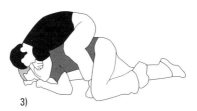

3)

Shooting the Hips Back with Combatives: If you cannot react with a leg counterattack or by sidestepping, you can shoot your hips back and lean your upper torso forward placing all your body weight on the attacker's head and upper torso. By sprawling backward keeping your weight on the balls of your feet and your feet spread wide, you create superior leverage, preventing the attacker from reaching your legs. He will fall face down, putting you in an advantageous position for counterattacks, including a knee to the head on elbow strike to the neck.

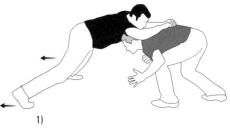

1)

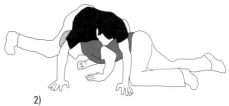

2)

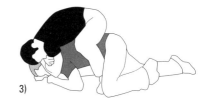

3)

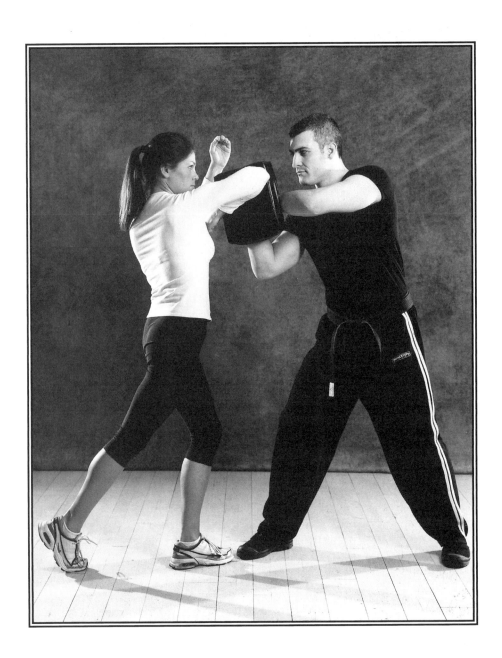

CHAPTER 7

Mastering Escapes

Learn how to extricate yourself
from grabs, holds, chokes, pulls,
and other dangerous situations

If your upper- and lower-body strikes fail to end a violent encounter, the situation can deteriorate quickly, with your attacker moving in and grabbing you. Once your attacker grabs you, he can inflict a life-threatening choke hold. Other types of close-contact grappling include hair pulling, headlocks, and bear hugs, all of which can put you in an extremely vulnerable position. In this chapter you will learn how to defend against these dangerous offensive techniques. Even if your attacker manages to work his arms around your neck and begins to choke you, you can still defend yourself with *krav maga!* Learning such defensive techniques against these types of hostile acts is crucial to making you proficient in the *krav maga* self-defense curriculum.

In this chapter you will learn many release techniques and defenses. They all operate on the same principles: fight back, build on your instincts, and use your attacker's momentum against him if possible. For example, if an opponent grabs one or both of your arms, strike back with your free arm, legs, and any other free body areas (even your forehead). As an attacker pulls you in one direction, enhance these counterattacks by moving in the same direction. This uses the attacker's momentum against him, allowing your punches, elbows, kicks, knees, and head butts to connect with greater force.

You may wish to release from a grab without resorting to combative strikes. Combative strikes are usually integral to a release from a grab. With or without strikes, to get your attacker to let go, find your attacker's grip's weakest angle and work against the thumb, the weakest digit. Do not, however, work against the combined strength of your opponent's remaining four clutched fingers. Arm-grab releases build the foundation for choke releases, which can extricate you from one of the most life-threatening methods of attack.

With enough practice you will begin to recognize where an opening is—that is, the spot on your attacker's grip where you can best use your technique to break a hold. To demonstrate this simple principle, bring your right thumb to your right index finger, creating a circle or an "okay" gesture. Insert your left thumb underneath and through the circle. If you had to create an opening in the circle with your left hand, you would not be able to do it by pushing against the web of your right hand. Rather, you would have to pull it against the tips of your thumb and forefinger, the weak link in the circle.

The same principle applies to breaking arm grabs and choke holds. You'll work against the thumb's weakest spot to pry the fingers apart and break your attacker's grip. In many techniques in this chapter, you will find the opening by *plucking* your attacker's hand or hands. With your cupped hand, you'll grab the attacker's hand or forearm from underneath and push or pull in the direction of the opening.

Before you learn any specific techniques, practice finding the opening. Ask a partner to grab your arm from the front, side, or rear while you are standing, sitting, or lying on your back. In each instance, notice your partner's grip and find the weakest link to break that grip. Below, you'll find a few variations and angles to practice.

1. Your partner grabs your left arm with his right. Grab your left hand with your right hand and, with your hands clasped together, pull your hands and arms toward the opening where your partner's thumb meets his fingers.

2. Your partner grabs your right arm with his right. Rotate your body away from your attacker (and toward the opening). You can also pluck the attacker's arm from underneath as you execute a release toward the opening.

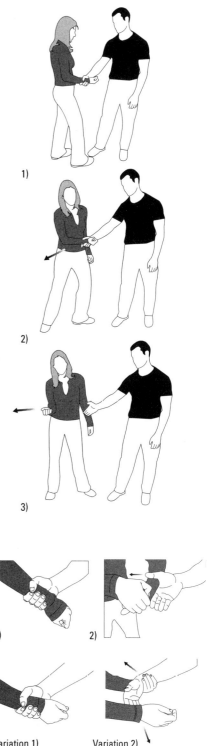

1)

2)

3)

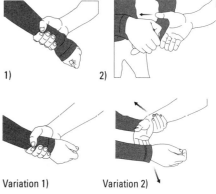

1)   2)

Variation 1)   Variation 2)

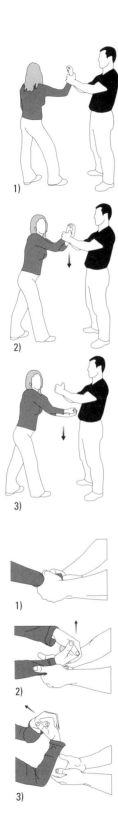

3. Your partner uses two arms to grab one of your wrists or forearms. Reach over the top of the grab and pull your hand toward your near ear, taking care not to hit yourself. You can also pluck the attacker's hand and execute the same technique as you did in situation 1 above by angling your arm movement toward you, working against the weakest part of your opponent's grip: his thumb and index finger.

4. Your partner uses two hands to grab one of your hands above your head. Reach underneath the grip and pull down on your arm that is being grabbed.

TRUE KRAVIST

A young woman trained in *krav maga* was walking down a crowded avenue in New York City when a man grabbed her bag. Reacting as she was taught, she moved with the assailant as he yanked at her bag and delivered a crippling sidekick to his knee. A nearby police officer saw the incident and ran over to make the arrest. While handcuffing the would-be purse snatcher, the officer commented, "Do you realize a little girl just beat you up!" The crowd that had gathered applauded.

5. Your partner grabs both of your arms at the wrists or forearms with both of his arms. Cross your arms and pull them toward you (toward the opening) as you kick and knee him until he lets go. Alternatively, you may rotate your forearms up, following a semicircular path to release. If the hold is high, rotate your arms down while taking a step back.

Defending a Purse or Briefcase Snatch

To defend yourself against common street snatching, move with your attacker and apply a flurry of strikes.

In this situation you have a few options. You can secure your purse or briefcase with one or both hands and move in the direction of the attacker's pull. As you move with the attacker's pull, employ *retzev* combatives such as a side kick to the knee followed by knees and elbows. Another option would be straight punches to your opponent's face and neck followed by utilizing your elbows and knees. A third option would be to whip or gouge the eyes followed by the combatives just described. (Of course, if you sense the situation could put you in physical jeopardy, you should simply release the bag.) You may also use the bag as a shield or even as a blunt weapon. Keep in mind that a large duffle bag or heavy backpack can encumber your movements. Although a backpack still allows your arms free movement, it will affect your movements, especially if it is heavy and you shift weight. A slung duffle bag's weight will affect your movements as well, but the weight will not be as evenly distributed, possibly resulting in an even greater hindrance.

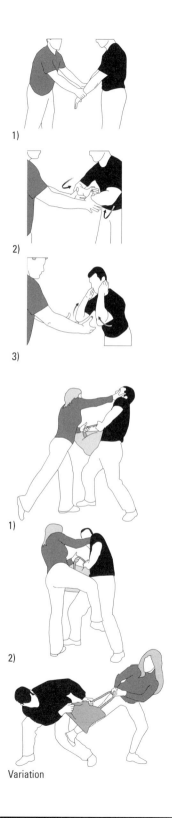

1)

2)

3)

1)

2)

Variation

Combative Strikes to Release from a Shirt Hold

Combative releases from shirt holds are just that: use your strike arsenal to target the attacker's vulnerable areas.

If the attacker pulls you, move in the direction of the pull and employ *retzev* combatives such as straight punches, knees, or eye gouges. If you do not feel your life is in danger, use gentler joint manipulation (such as the finger techniques manipulation from chapter 4) that are not designed to produce damage to your opponent.

Front Choke-Hold Release

A choke can quickly render you unconscious or worse. Yet as long as you can still breathe, you can fight back. Krav maga choke defenses build on instinct and are particularly illustrative of Imi's practical approach to self-defense. Most people, for example, will reach for their throats when choking on a piece of food. Similarly, if a garment is too tight around your neck, you will automatically pull down on the constricting material to give yourself breathing room.

Bury your chin into your chest while keeping your eyes up to maintain your vision. This cuts off access to your throat and makes it more difficult for your attacker to get his hands around your neck. From here, you have a number of options, as described in the following defenses.

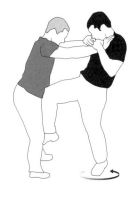

Front choke-defense 1. Tuck your chin and cup both of your hands in front of your face. Curl your fingers in and together to produce two hooks with your hands. To remove an attacker's hands from your throat, use a short outward plucking motion with your hands against the attacker's weakest digit: the thumbs. Do not actually pluck the thumbs. Rather, with a clawlike grip, pluck underneath the thumb where the thumb joint meets the hand. Rest your hands (and your attacker's hands) at the top of your chest muscles. By trapping the attacker's hands to your upper chest just below your clavicle, you eliminate the threat of another attack from his hands. Add a simultaneous front knee and you have your preliminary front choke defense. Follow up with multiple knees, elbows, gouges, and other *retzev* counterattacks.

Front choke-defense 2. Use this defense when your legs and knees are not available to counterattack, for example, if an attacker chokes you from across a table. With your left hand, pluck the attacker's right hand as you pivot forward on your right leg and gouge your attacker's eyes with your right hand. This pivot also adds a body defense by turning your neck away from the attacker's grasp. Your right arm must shoot up between the attacker's arms to attack his eyes, not to the outside of his arms. This inside counterattack gives you direct access to the attacker's face and little opportunity for him to block your counterattacks. Follow up with an instantaneous straight knee to the groin with your right leg. Your base leg will probably slide a bit (known in Hebrew as *glicha*) to accommodate your straight knee to the attacker's groin. If the opponent's groin is too far away for a knee

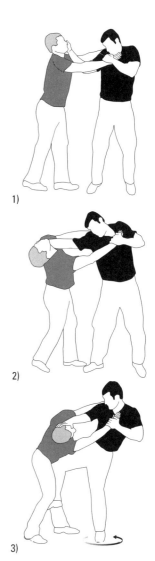

1)

2)

3)

TRUE KRAVIST

A woman observed the end of a *krav maga* class. She asked the instructor what she could learn in five minutes. The instructor taught her two moves: a thumb gouge to the eye and a groin strike with the same side knee. The next night a stalker attacked her and threw her to the ground. Using the attacker's cheek as a guide, she gouged him in the eye and kneed him in the groin. She escaped and the police later identified the attacker by the damage to his eye.

strike, simply extend your lower leg out, making groin contact with any point on your lower leg. Follow up with additional *retzev* combatives such as elbows, gouges, uppercut punches, and body strikes.

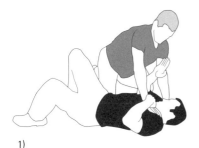

1)

Choke Release from the Ground with the Attacker to Your Side

If an attacker chokes you from a side position while on his knees, he can exert great pressure by leaning his body into the choke. A modification of choke-defense 2 will release the choke hold.

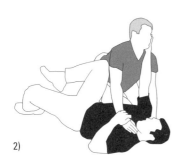

2)

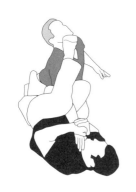

3)

Use this defense when the attacker is to your side (in this case, the right side) on his knees and your back is against the ground. Use your left hand to pluck your attacker's right hand and launch an inside attack (between the attacker's arms) with your other arm to the attacker's eye, jaw, or throat as you transfer your weight to your other shoulder. (Note: if your attacker is to your left, you will pluck with your right-outside hand and counterattack with your left-inside hand.) Follow up with a diagonal knee strike with your closest knee, the right knee (in this example) to the opponent's side, striking him in the ribs. After you make contact, keep the knee moving until your shin presses against the attacker's side. (If flexibility is a problem, do the best that you can. If you cannot reach the attacker's side with your knee, you can resort to body strikes, but try to keep the attacker's outside arm pinned.) Once your shin is in place, extend yourself as far away from the attacker as you can, but do not release his outside arm just yet. By creating separation but not letting go of the attacker, you can deliver a modified-defensive front kick to his head with your other (outside) leg. The power behind this kick will likely knock him backward. You can follow up with additional kicks, including a short hammer kick by slamming your heel down on your opponent and continuing your *retzev* counterattacks.

Choke Release from the Ground with the Attacker Straddling You

If an attacker chokes you from a straddling position (also known as the mounted position), he'll be able to push his upper body down on your throat, creating greater pressure. You can still, however, extricate yourself from this seemingly grim situation.

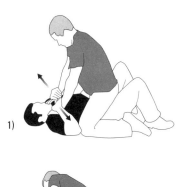

1)

Tuck your chin and use the same upper-body technique as choke-release 1, but modify it to include a hip buck to get your attacker off you. To buck your hips, you must raise them up and to one side to throw the attacker. Practice this buck by lying flat on the ground with your legs bent and feet on the ground. Rotate your body to one side by raising one shoulder off the ground, transferring your weight to your other shoulder. Your feet will move to accommodate your turning movement. You should be able to launch the attacker provided he has not hooked his heels into your sides. Once you have thrown him, you are in a strong position to hit your opponent repeatedly in the groin. If you cannot launch him, attack with strikes to the groin, midsection, neck, face, as well as elbows to his thighs, launching him whenever and however you can.

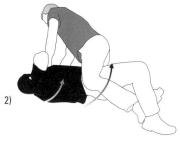

2)

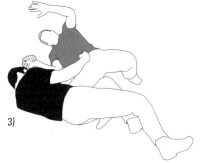

3)

Choke Release from the Ground with the Attacker Between Your Legs

Use this defense if an attacker tries to choke you when positioned between your legs while on his knees (or if he is attempting to position himself there). You can employ this technique before the attacker attempts to grab your neck. You can also use it to defend yourself against a sexual assault.

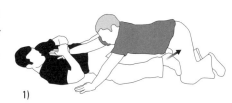

1)

Tuck in your chin. Use the same upper-body technique as in choke-release 1 with this slight modification. Slide backward away from the attacker and kick the attacker in the groin. As you kick, turn your toes to the outside so that the foot is parallel to the ground. Continue with various strikes as openings present themselves. Escape as soon as possible.

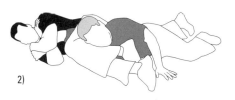

2)

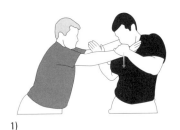

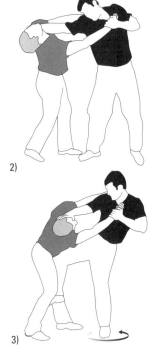

Side-Choke Release

Use this technique if an attacker chokes you with his hands while he is positioned to your side.

This defensive technique is a modification of front choke-defense 2. In a side-choke defense, always pluck with the hand farthest away from your attacker and counterattack with the near arm. The attacker's front arm grasping the front of your neck presents the most serious danger. While it may not be pleasant to have the attacker's hand on the back of your neck, a counterattack to the opponent's eye, throat, or groin must take precedence over the hand on the back of your neck. After the initial defense, follow-through with *retzev* counterattacks, such as knees, elbows, and any other opportune combative. The opponent will probably release your neck at this point.

Circumstances might place the attacker in close proximity to your side. In this case use the pluck; however, due to the attacker's close distance, your counterattack strike will now target the groin. Cup your hand and slap at the attacker's groin by rotating your wrist out, slapping up at the testicles with your cupped fingers. Follow up with an upward elbow to the chin or throat and other strikes.

Rear Choke Release While Pulled from Behind

Use this defense if an attacker chokes you from behind while pulling you backward.

Tuck in your chin, dip your shoulder, and turn instantaneously into your opponent. Deliver a devastating counterattack, such as a punch to the throat with the arm opposite your turning shoulder. See Defense Against a Stranglehold with a Rope.

Defense Against a Stranglehold with a Rope

If someone is trying to strangle you with a rope, belt, or a wire, you have precious little time to react.

Tuck your chin, dip your shoulder, and turn instantaneously into your opponent. Deliver a devastating counterattack, such as a punch to the throat with the arm opposite your turning shoulder.

Front Choke Release While the Attacker Pushes Forward

An assailant can choke you from the front while pushing you with enough force to send you backward. If taken off balance by a forward push or choke, your natural tendency will be to take a step backward to regain your balance. The corresponding krav maga *technique, once again, builds on your natural reaction and will allow you to maintain your balance while positioning you to defend the choke.*

As you take a definitive step back with your left foot to regain your balance, clear the choke by bringing your right arm to your right ear with your elbow bent 90 degrees so that your forearm is flush with the top of your head, with your biceps touching your ear. Using this arm positioning, pivot at least 90 degrees to clear your opponent's hands as you pluck and trap one or both of the opponent's arms. Follow up with an outside chop by whacking at the opponent's throat with your forearm or underside of a clenched fist on a parallel plane to the ground. Follow up with knee and elbow strikes, along with other *retzev* techniques, depending on the distance between you and your attacker.

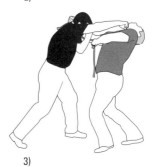

1)

2)

3)

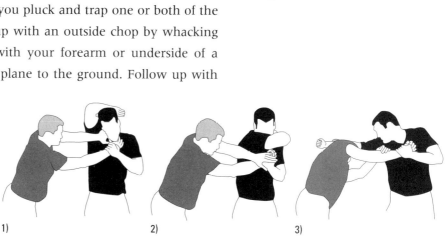

1)   2)   3)

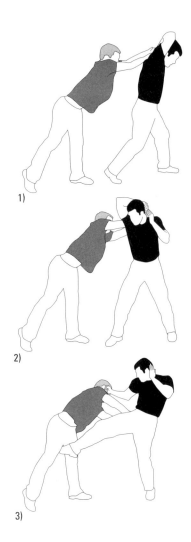

1)

2)

3)

Rear Choke Release While the Attacker Pushes Forward

An assailant can unexpectedly choke you with enough force from behind to push you forward. If taken off balance, your natural tendency will be to step forward. As in the front choke, the corresponding krav maga *technique for a pushing rear choke builds on your natural reaction to maintain your balance while positioning you to defend the choke.*

You'll take a definitive forward step to regain your balance and while tucking your chin use a similar clearing motion as the previous technique. Step forward with your left foot and bring your right arm to your ear with your elbow bent 90 degrees. Your forearm is flush with the top of your head, and your bicep is touching your ear. Using this arm positioning, spin around 180 degrees toward the side of your upraised arm to face your attacker. This action will clear both of the attacker's arms from your throat. After pivoting through to clear the threat of your attacker's arms, follow up with counterattacks, such as a hammer strike and then knee or kick with your near leg to your attacker's groin, followed by other *retzev* combatives.

Side Headlock Release

The side headlock can jolt your neck and place you in a vulnerable position. This attack is common and often demonstrated on the playground. Your attacker can drop his weight to the ground to exert great force on your neck while forcing you down with him. Alternatively, the attacker can torque your neck, causing serious harm. The attacker could also punch you in the face repeatedly with his opposite arm or drive your head into a wall. As with all defenses, the best defense against a headlock is to avoid being put into one.

Reacting at the earliest possible moment is crucial. Assume the side headlock attack comes from your left. Therefore, the attacker is positioned near your left shoulder and most likely in front of you. If you see the headlock coming, tuck in your chin and turn it slightly to the left. Then wage a preemptive defense by bracing your left arm across the opponent's neck or face, attacking the eyeball. Bring your left arm behind the attacker's back and over his right shoulder to hook his eye with your most convenient finger while simultaneously using your right arm to deliver slaps to the groin using a cupped hand. (Another option is use your middle and index fingers to reach under the attacker's nose and drive it straight back or grab hair to leverage the head back.)

If possible, prevent the attacker from clasping his hands together by timing your defense correctly or, alternatively, using your right arm to stop his lower hand from grasping his other arm. Proceed with the groin attack. This will work effectively against most people; however, some people can withstand this pressure and will continue their attack. Bring the attacker's head back by pushing into his eye socket, exposing his neck to strikes. You may use an inside chop with the underside of your hand or a clenched fist swung into the target on a parallel plane to the ground, punch, or any other form of attack from your free arm.

If you are placed in a headlock on the ground with the opponent to your side, use the same defense with this modification. Turn away from the attacker's arm underneath your neck. As you do so, apply pressure against your attacker's eyeball or filtrum with one hand while striking the exposed groin with the other hand, forcing the attacker to release.

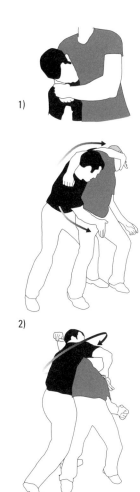

1)

2)

3)

Front Headlock or "Guillotine" Release

The front headlock or "guillotine" hold can wrench your neck, choke you, or do worse. In this type of headlock or choke, an opponent facing you has taken one of his arms and wrapped it around your neck from the outside. In other words, if an opponent is placing you in this hold with his right arm underneath your neck, he has come from your right side (his left side), pulling you down toward him to secure your neck by clasping his

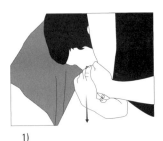

1)

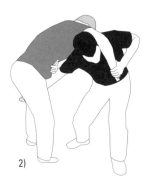

2)

right arm with his left arm. In addition, your attacker can fall to the ground in a pincerlike motion with his weight pulling up on your neck to exert great force to choke you or severely damage your neck.

Let's assume the attacker has his right arm around the back of your neck and under your chin/neck area. Tuck your chin into your chest and turn your chin to face the attacker's clasped hands. With both of your arms, locate and grasp the attacker's forearm that he is trying to insert under your chin. Yank down with all of your might on the attacker's forearm, positioning your hands as close as possible to his interlocked hands. Clear the arm forcefully from your chin/neck area. Turn your right shoulder into the opponent to help create separation, continue to yank down on the attacker's forearm with your left hand, and use your right hand to execute multiple attacks to the groin with a cupped hand or fist. Once you have "loosened" the attacker up, continue to hold his right forearm. Step with your right leg underneath his right armpit, keeping his right arm firmly secured. Do not let go. After stepping underneath to clear yourself from the attack, keep the right arm pinned and deliver additional *retzev* counterattacks.

Forearm Choke Release from Behind

Forearm chokes (also called blood chokes) from the rear are some of the most effective and dangerous strangulation techniques. They can crush your windpipe or cut off the blood flow from the carotid arteries to the brain. These are powerful chokes because the attacker's entire body can be maneuvered to exert maximum force while you are in a precarious defensive position. You must react instantaneously to these highly effective offensive techniques.

Let's assume the attacker has his right arm under your chin/neck area. Tuck your chin and turn it slightly in the direction of the attacker's interlocked hands. In any kind of forearm choke, as in the front headlock, always turn toward the side where the attacker's hands are clasped. If you do not turn this way you will be turning into the attacker's bent elbow where there is no opening.

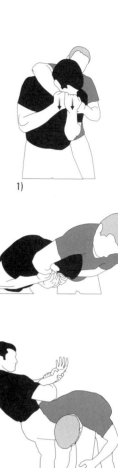

1)

Simultaneously, with both of your hands, locate and grasp the attacker's forearm that he is trying to insert under your chin. Yank down with both of your arms, with your hands as close as possible to his interlocked hands. Clear the arm forcefully from your chin/neck area. As soon as you create separation, dip your left shoulder and step backward with your left leg while wheeling your right shoulder in the direction of your attacker's right shoulder. Continue to step through and underneath the attacker's right armpit while holding the attacker's arm firmly pincered against your body with both of your arms. Immediately deliver a knee from your rear leg to the attacker's exposed midsection, followed by other *retzev* counterattacks.

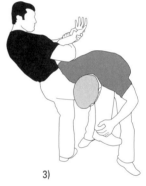

2)

If you cannot release immediately from the blood choke from the rear, revert to a modified-side-headlock release, but, do not release your arms from the attacker's forearm until you can breathe enough to execute the side-headlock release. This modified release keeps your inside (left) arm exerting as much resistance as you can on the attacker's forearm under your chin to alleviate the pressure. While keeping forceful resistance on your opponent's choking arm with your initial defense, turn into the attacker with your outside (right) leg and deliver multiple attacks to his groin. Once you have "loosened up" your opponent, you have the option of your regular side headlock release.

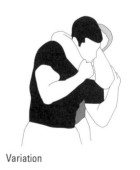

3)

Note: A "professional" variation of the blood-choke hold involves the attacker applying one arm underneath your chin while snaking the other arm around the back of your head and gripping his own bicep. This is a strong hold, especially when the attacker draws back with the choking arm while pressing forward with the rear arm against the back of the head. The choke release is similar to that discussed previously; however, you must take your same-side arm as the attacker is reaching behind your head and yank it at the biceps muscle to dislodge the grip. Your other arm yanks down on the forearm below your chin.

Variation

Yet another variation of the rear and blood-choke releases might involve an assailant grabbing you from behind with one hand covering your mouth and the other arm gripping your far-side arm. To release, pluck the hand from your mouth and turn toward your assailant, toward your arm the attacker is securing. In other words, you are plucking in one direction and pivoting your body toward your assailant in the other direction.

Forearm Choke Release While on the Ground

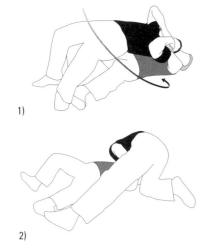

1)

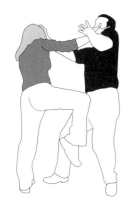

2)

When grappling on the ground, an attacker may try to put you in a blood choke while he is behind you. Good ground fighters will pincer their legs around you to prevent your escape and extend their bodies to strengthen the choke or face bar.

Do *not* let an opponent wrap his legs around from underneath, especially with his chest to your back. Intercept his legs with your own legs as he attempts to pincer you. This requires bringing your legs up to ward off the pincer. Use the same chin tuck and two-hand pluck release as described for other forearm releases, except this time you must bridge the body by raising your body on the balls of your feet and rolling under the arm to pin it. Then follow up with *retzev* combatives.

Hair-Pull Defenses from the Front

If an opponent pulls your hair, he can control your head, wrench your neck, and cause acute pain. The danger from a hair pull comes from the head being immobilized or forced in the direction of an attack. For example, an attacker can grab your hair to drive your head into a knee strike or to smash your face into an object, such as a wall or table.

To understand how to extricate yourself from a hair pull, you must first know how to execute one. To exert maximum pressure and control of the head, spread your fingers and shoot them through the hair at the base of the scalp. Once you have ample hair between your fingers, make a tight fist. Now you can pull the head in any number of directions.

To get out of a hair pull, do not yank your head in the opposite direction of the attacker's pull. Rather, move with him to use his momentum against him while also easing your physical discomfort. Go on the offensive immediately by moving toward your attacker, in the direction you are being pulled. Clamp the heel of one palm against the back of your attacker's pulling hand while executing immediate counterattacks, such as strikes to the face and throat, eye gouges, and kicks to the groin. To reiterate, do not pull your head in the opposite direction to resist the attacker's pull.

If your attacker has tried to grab your hair to pull your head into his knee, apply the 360-degree instinctive-defense position 7 downward forearm (see p. 58) while executing counterattacks to the groin, followed by additional *retzev* combatives.

Hair-Pull Defenses from the Nearside

As with the front hair pull, the defense against a hair pull from the nearside requires you to move in the direction of the pull.

You have several options for your counterattack, including elbowing your opponent in the ribcage, followed by *retzev* counterattacks. You may also close the distance to your attacker with a slap to the groin with your near hand or wheel into your opponent to attack the groin with your far hand, followed by additional combatives. A last alternative is to move into the attacker and use a variation of the headlock defense from the side. Finish with *retzev* combatives.

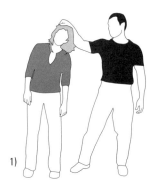

1)

Hair-Pull Defenses from the Far Side

Use this technique if your attacker reaches around your head to your far side to pull you quickly toward him.

Your defense is similar to the hair-pull defense from the near-side except that you must turn into the attacker to slap his groin. Finish with *retzev* counterattacks.

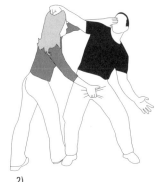

2)

Hair-Pull Defenses from the Rear

Use this defense, similar to defending a pulling choke from the rear, if an attacker grabs your hair from behind and yanks back hard. People with long hair, especially hair braided or in ponytails, are particularly suscep-tible to this type of attack. Do not resist the attack by leaning forward against the pull.

Move in the direction of the pull with a pivot to face your at-tacker. A pull from behind will require you to pivot 180 degrees and dip your shoulder to face the attacker. This will alleviate the tension on your scalp. Your turn must involve a simultaneous at-tack, preferably to the attacker's groin, throat, or head, followed by additional combatives.

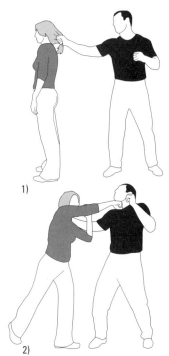

1)

2)

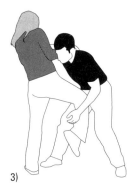

3)

Defense Against a Head Butt

If your attacker slams the hardest part of his head—the forehead—into your face, especially your nose, he can inflict serious damage.

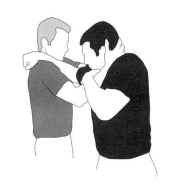

Place a forearm brace across your opponent's throat by using a diagonal stance to the attacker where your elbow is bent approximately 90 degrees. Your right shoulder is directly across from the attacker's right shoulder with your forearm planted across his throat. Notice that this body positioning prevents the opponent from reaching you with a head butt, but allows you to reach him. Take him down with various strikes.

You can also place your elbow in the end position of either your horizontal or vertical elbow to the face. Another option is the educational defense discussed in chapter 4, placing pressure against the opponent's trachea. An opponent will be hard-pressed to initiate a head-butt action while in this position.

Front Bear-Hug Defenses with the Arms Free

A face-to-face torso grab or "bear hug" can crush your ribs or pick your entire body up and smash it to the ground. Your opponent may grab underneath your arms, allowing them to go free, or may pin them to your sides.

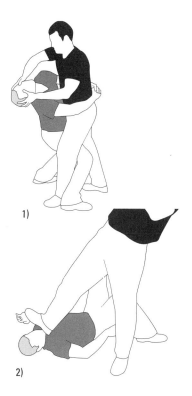

1)

The best defense against this and other high-grabbing or throwing attacks is to preempt them with a long-range kick or knee to the opponent's groin or midsection or medium-range straight punch. If you do get caught up in a bear hug, however, and your arms are free, you have several options. Attack your opponent's face, including thumbs to the eyes or underneath the nose, and other strikes to the face. You may also be able to knee your attacker in the groin and midsection. Combine these techniques with an outside leg hook (see chapter 6) and you have a potent defense. Combine to neutralize the threat with stomps, kicks, and additional *retzev* combatives.

2)

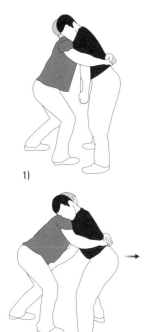

1)

2)

3)

Front Bear-Hug Defenses with the Arms Pinned

Bear-hug-type holds can give an attacker a dominant position, especially if your arms are pinned—but not if you employ the proper defensive techniques immediately!

Shoot your hips back about six inches, giving yourself enough room to simultaneously insert your hands in front of your body to strike the attacker's groin. At the same time, bring your head to one side and tuck your chin into your neck to protect against an inadvertent head butt by your opponent. (A slap to your opponent's groin will likely bring his head forward). After multiple groin strikes, reach with both hands behind the opponent, and, using a hand pinch (grabbing and making a tight fist), grab clothing, flesh, or both, and continue with knee strikes. You can also bite the opponent's neck and continue with additional strikes.

Low-Front Bear Hug with the Arms Free or Arms Pinned

A low-front bear hug can be difficult to distinguish from a tackle. A tackle usually involves a running start, enabling the tackler to drive his body into your body, taking you backward to the ground. The low-bear-hug lifts and throws or squeezes the torso strongly.

If you are attacked with a low-front bear hug and your arms are free, target the face with upper body strikes and knee your attacker in the groin, midsection, or solar plexus. You can shoot your hips back and deliver a vertical elbow to the nape of the neck, followed by *retzev* counterattacks. If your arms are pinned, use the same defense you learned against a high bear hug but lower your body for your defensive moves.

Rear-Bear-Hug Defense with Your Arms Free

A close-grab "bear hug" from the rear places you in great danger of being driven forward into a wall or the ground or being thrown.

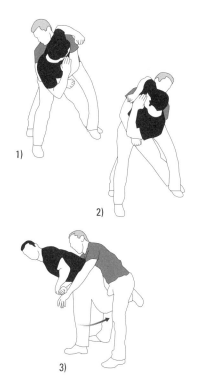

Drop your weight and, if possible, shoot one of your legs backward to hook your opponent's leg from the inside. Hook the back of your opponent's Achilles tendon with the crook of your ankle and foot to prevent him from lifting you. A split moment after you drop your weight, begin your counterattack with numerous rear horizontal elbow strikes, alternating from one side to the other rapidly. If your opponent sways his upper body one way, you will catch him in the opposite direction with this flurry of alternating elbows.

You can also counterstrike with an upward "mule" kick by striking your heel into the attacker's groin. Another option is to lift one leg and smash your attacker's shin with the side of the upraised foot and then rake your foot down the attacker's shin and stomp down on his foot. To ensure the opponent releases his hands, strike the back of his top clasped hand repeatedly as you would rap on a door. Turn and face your attacker to continue *reztev* counterattacks.

Rear-Bear-Hug Defenses with Your Arms Pinned

A close-grab "bear hug" from the rear places you in great danger of being driven forward into a wall or the ground or being thrown, especially if your arms are pinned.

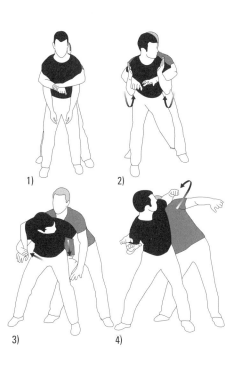

If you are attacked from behind with a rear bear hug and your attacker pins your arms to your side, drop your weight and, if possible, insert of one of your legs between the opponent's legs, hooking your opponent's same-side leg from the inside. As you drop your weight, shoot your hands upward to loosen the attacker's grip. If the attacker's arms release, continue with the same rear-bear-hug defense you learned above with the arms free, along with multiple-rear elbow and groin strikes, a mule kick to the groin with your inside leg, and stomps to your opponent's feet. If he does not fully release, slide side to side while executing groin strikes with hammer fists. Finish with *retzev* counterattacks.

If the attacker's arms do not release, shift your body weight to one side or the other. This will expose the attacker's groin. Look behind you and slap at the attacker's groin. Rapidly shift your weight to the other side if you cannot hit the groin on the first attempt. Shifting your body weight, utilizing the strength of your lower body, and taking short, emphatic steps will loosen the attacker's hold to allow your counterattack.

Defenses Against Bear Hugs from the Side

An opponent can use a bear hug from the side to drive you sideways. Your arms may be free or pinned.

If your arms are free, you can use a similar defense learned previously for the bear hug with your arms free: gouging the opponent's eyes while hooking your nearside leg to the outside of his nearside leg to drive him backward. (You can also shoot the hips back.) Finish with stomps and additional *retzev* counterattacks.

If your arms are pinned, use a similar defense to what you would use against a bear hug from the front with your arms pinned. Create distance with your nearside shoulder by shifting your hips back, keeping your head to one side, and delivering a simultaneous groin attack with your hands, followed by additional counterattacks.

Bear-Hug Defenses While Being Lifted

Your chances of being lifted will be greatly reduced if you insert one of your legs inside one of the attacker's legs. Should the attacker succeed in lifting you with a bear hug, your defenses will remain the same with a few modifications. This is a particularly important technique for women to master, as their lighter weight makes them more likely to be lifted.

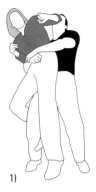

1)

Hook one of your outside legs tightly around your opponent's outside leg. If you are lifted from the front and your arms are free, you may do the same as in the first bear-hug defense using the arms-free eye gouge. Finish with *retzev* counterattacks. A double-handed slap to the opponent's ears is also effective ("boxing the ears").

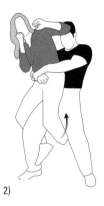

2)

If you are lifted from the front and your arms are pinned, hook one leg and use the other leg to deliver knee strikes. You may also be in a position to use hand strikes to the groin, or, if necessary, bite the attacker's neck. Finish with *retzev* counterattacks.

If your arms are free, hook your outside leg tightly to your opponent's outside leg and proceed as you would with either the arms free or arms pinned rear-bear-hug defenses. Consider a mule kick to the groin as well. Finish with *retzev* counterattacks.

If your arms are pinned, hook your outside leg tightly around your opponent's leg and use the low-front bear hug with the arms-free or arms-pinned defense. Finish with *retzev* counterattacks.

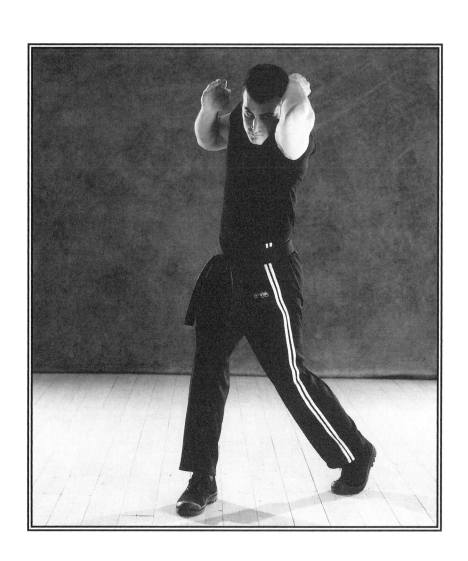

CHAPTER 8

Your Personal *Krav Maga*

Build Your Fitness and Fighting Skills
with Regular Practice

Now that you know *krav maga*'s basic techniques, it's time to put them together into a comprehensive fitness and self-defense program. It's one thing to understand the techniques. It's quite another to know them intuitively. In chapters 4 through 8, you learned how to punch, kick, knee, gouge, and generally defend yourself against an attacker. In this and the following chapter, you'll learn how to effectively pair various techniques into an effective fighting—and fitness—strategy.

In this chapter you'll learn the principles behind pairing punches with kicks, knees with elbows, and so on. You'll learn how to design your own unique and intuitive set of self-defense movements. In chapter 9 you'll find a twelve-week training plan that will not only get you in fighting shape (possibly the best shape of your life) but also help you to practice the techniques and drills until they become instinctive and natural. That way, whenever you find yourself in a threatening situation, you'll be able to react automatically—without thinking or hesitating. You'll respond with the techniques that you have practiced, in the sequences in which you practiced them. By the end of the program, you'll be able to successfully defend yourself in any situation.

Before embarking on the twelve-week program, let's first take a look at the philosophy behind the techniques. Follow these pointers whenever you find yourself in a dangerous situation.

Walk away. Just because you know how to defend yourself from an attack doesn't mean that you need to prove it. If you can walk away safely from a potential confrontation, do it. Don't allow your ego to put you in harm's way. Similarly, respond with the appropriate level of force.

Select more passive techniques for less-threatening situations. For example, certain hand and shirt releases can disengage you from a threatening grab and create enough separation for you to run away. If the threat is slightly more serious and you cannot get away, ratchet up the techniques one level by applying a joint-lock or submission hold, causing the attacker discomfort but no temporary or permanent damage. If you feel your life is in danger, however, take the same techniques an additional rung higher on the use-of-force ladder by using punishing strikes and joint dislocations, resulting in temporary or permanent damage.

If you must react, stay on the offensive. Once you recognize a potential threat, assume control of the situation as quickly as possible. If your opponent is preparing to punch or kick you, strike first by kicking him in the groin before he launches the strike. Do not wait to be attacked. You may have to perform not just one defensive movement to ward off an attack, but, at the soonest possible moment, you must transition to the offensive and stay on the attack using your own combinations.

Switch techniques if your initial strategy fails. If a combative fails against your first body target, switch your attack to secondary body targets.

Assess your surroundings. Be aware of your advantages and disadvantages in a potential fight situation. Survey your surroundings to determine what you can use to your advantage, including the nearest escape route.

Dictate the fight using *retzev* combatives. Use the motto "Expect the unexpected" to your advantage by implementing continuous and fluid *retzev* counterattacks in different combinations and strategies designed to take your assailant off guard. Neutralize the threat without hesitation by seamlessly switching from a defense to an overwhelming offense. Dictate the fight yourself.

Never accept defeat or surrender. If you can breathe, you can fight. Do not accept the notion of defeat. Do what you must to prevail. Fight to survive—and to win.

Keep moving. You can keep your attacker off guard by switching body positions as well as the rhythm and nature of your attacks and counterattacks. Near-constant movement on your part will also help you find the most advantageous position, either to your opponent's dead side or in a location that allows you to strike through an opening your opponent has created. As you move, however, avoid turning your back to the attacker, especially when you are close to each other.

Use the right strike for the right fighting distance. Different types of strikes will work more or less effectively depending on your distance from your opponent. *Krav maga* categorizes a fight in four ranges: long (a leg's distance away or farther), intermediate (an arm's length apart), short (half an arm's length apart), and close (grappling distance). Ideally, you can initiate and, perhaps, end the confrontation from the longest distance using your most powerful tools: your legs. If you cannot neutralize the threat at this range, however, close the distance and take further *retzev* action.

Below you'll find the best techniques to use for each fighting distance:

Long. Focus your technique on movements that use the legs, which house the body's strongest muscles. If you recognize an impending threat early enough, you can kick your attacker, using your legs to keep him farthest from your danger zone.

Intermediate. Strike at your attacker with your arms and hands. Use quick punches or elongated hand strikes.

Short. Your attacker is now too close to effectively punch, which necessitates using your elbows and knees as weapons. Fortunately, these two joints are incredibly durable and hard surfaces.

Close. Now that you and your attacker are grappling, you may find it difficult to punch, kick, or knee him. You still, however, have many options. You can bite, choke, and gouge your attacker. You can also apply joint dislocation and breaking techniques. Sometimes going to the ground should be your last choice. This is especially true if there are multiple opponents within the vicinity who could attack you simultaneously. Once on the ground, return to your feet as soon as practical.

Do not play to your opponent's strengths. Use techniques that counter your opponent's strengths, especially when an opponent's training is evident. For example, when fighting with a much taller opponent, negate his superior reach by moving in close. If your opponent is shorter and your limbs are longer, use your superior reach with longer range strikes to keep him away.

Look for vulnerabilities and use your more competent techniques. If you cannot walk or run away from the encounter, keep as safe a distance as possible, especially if your attacker is trying to move in. When fighting off an attacker, start with the long-distance techniques (kicks) first, which will help create space between you and the attacker. If the attacker successfully moves closer, then opt for intermediate-distance technique (punches), followed by short-distance (elbows and knees) techniques, and finishing close as a last resort. Elbows and knees are always a strong finish. If your attacker, however, is comfortable fighting with long-distance techniques, you'll want to eliminate this advantage by closing the distance as you continue the fight. Move to an infight using short punches, knees, elbows, head butts, catches, and throws. Conversely, to disengage from such close fighting, you must defend against punches, kicks, knees, elbows, clinches, head butts, and grabs with counterattacks that will create separation.

Read your opponent's next move before he makes it. Your opponent's stance or body positioning can often signal his offensive intentions and capabilities. For example, if your opponent is moving his hands like a boxer, you will likely face a flurry of punches. If your opponent drops into a low crouch with his hands positioned like a wrestler, you are probably facing a ground fighter. Obviously there are many variables, and not all fighting styles are a dead giveaway; however, if you learn to anticipate your opponent's next move, you can counterattack more effectively. Here are some ways you can counter various types of fighters:

BOXERS. Employ full-extension low kicks, which will prevent the boxer from getting close enough to use his hands. In addition, the boxer may not be trained to defend against this type of technique. You can also clinch a boxer but watch out for uppercuts and body shots and take him down for *retzev* groundwork to negate his punching ability.

GROUND FIGHTERS. This attacker will try to take you to the ground. Resist by using a series of combatives, releases, and evasive defenses, such as not letting your arm be grabbed for a lock or preventing the ground fighter from mounting you, especially from behind.

KICKERS. Someone displaying high kicks is more likely comfortable fighting from a distance. Move in and fight close. Bursting inside to close the distance will allow you to get inside the danger of these types of kicks through "infighting," using short combatives, such as elbows and knees and groundwork if necessary.

LEARN THE *KRAV MAGA* CHESS GAME. Just as a chess player thinks a number of moves ahead, so should you as a *kravist*. I strongly recommend you practice with a partner. This will help you to understand the body's movements, particularly how the body may or may not react to combatives against it. For example, a knee to an opponent's groin or midsection will double him over, leaving the back of his neck exposed for additional combatives or his face open to a knee-level strike. A thumb inserted into the eye socket will drive the head back, exposing the neck and bringing the groin forward for a knee strike. The more you understand your opponent's natural reaction to your movements, the more you'll be able to think ahead and plan your series of attacks and defenses with precision and insight.

ALWAYS FOLLOW UP WITH A SERIES OF COUNTERSTRIKES. Once you have become fluent with one technique, combine it with others into a flowing sequence. For example, after learning straight punches with both arms, try combining the left and right punches in rapid succession. After mastering straight punches and knee strikes, combine your left- and right-punch combination with knee strikes. Continuing further, try adding an elbow strike after the knee to create a four-part series and so on. Thus, you'll begin to create an instinctive and fluid *retzev* ("continuous motion") that you can call upon at any time. In the training plan in chapter 9, you'll complete a series of drills that will help you to develop *retzev*.

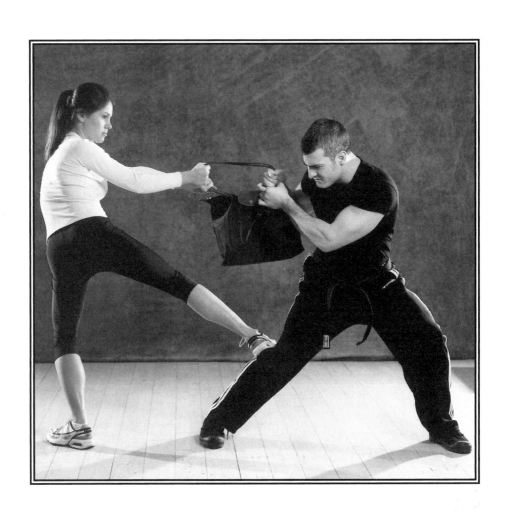

CHAPTER 9

The *Krav Maga* Combative Training Plan

Hone your skills, improve your fitness, and become a *kravist*

Welcome to the *kravist* training plan, a twelve-week program designed to take you from elbow shy to fighting fit. For this program you will practice the *krav maga* techniques for one hour per training session, three to four sessions a week. Some of your practice sessions will include a partner, and some you can complete alone. For some, I recommend you complete your drills in front of a mirror. For others I'll recommend you complete them with your eyes closed to better hone your instincts.

With practice and hard work, you can attain a high level of proficiency. Although it takes many years of study to become an expert under the Israeli curriculum, you can gain street proficiency against the most common unarmed confrontations—and get fighting fit—in about twelve weeks.

What Type of *Kravist* Have You Become? ⟵

If you practice consistently and diligently at least three to four hours a week with this training program, you will cover the core techniques for the first two belt levels, yellow and orange (see page 25). As you practice, your proficiency will improve. Here's what you can expect at each level of proficiency. The expert level takes many years to attain.

Level I: Novice   At the novice level, your reactions to conflict are still conscious. You must still deliberate your reactions, which have not yet become instinctive. Conditioned reflexive responses are not yet a part of the novice's arsenal. Movements are not fluid. For example, when defeating a choke from the front, a Level I trainee will pause briefly to analyze the situation before reacting, recall the appropriate technique, and then execute the technique. The Level I reaction is not yet instinctive but is on its way to becoming so.

Level II: Advanced   You reach this level when your subconscious assumes control. You now can respond instinctively to any threat and quickly assume control over the situation. When confronted with danger, you automatically respond as you have practiced or visualized. At this level, you are approaching a high degree of proficiency. In the same example of defending a choke from the front, a Level II trainee will react instantaneously by removing the attacker's hands and executing simultaneous counterattacks.

Level III: Expert   This expert level of the *kravist* requires innate reactions and movements. Muscle reaction and controlled movement take over the millisecond you assess and recognize a threat, allowing you to seamlessly execute your reaction. You will recall a scenario you have mentally stored through practice and visualization, and explode into action without the slightest hesitation. An expert Level III *kravist* will recognize that same impending choke attack before it happens—for example, by delivering a swift, offensive kick to the attacker's groin, or avoid the violent situation altogether.

⟵

Your Warm-Up and Cool-Down

Warm up before every practice session by gradually elevating your heart rate. This will prepare the muscles, joints, respiratory, and circulatory systems for your activity. First, you should increase your blood circulation with moderate cardiovascular activity, such as a light run, using an exercise bike, jumping jacks, jumping rope, or the like, for a minimum of ten minutes.

After you warm up, stretch gently to prepare your muscles, ligaments, and tendons for quick, explosive movements and maximum extension. Allow your body to gradually adjust to exertion and strain. Begin with stretching your neck and work your way down the body to your ankles and toes. You can do your own stretches or follow the sample stretching routine below. Hold each stretch for a count of ten, using "one-one-thousand, two-one-thousand . . . ten-one-thousand." Repeat each stretch on the left and right sides of your body.

The Neck   Gently rotate your neck to the left and then to the right in a circular motion. Then turn your head to look to your left, over your left shoulder, and to the right. Then look up and down.

The Shoulders   Gently shrug your shoulders both forward and back. Then rotate your arms forward in large circles, gradually tightening the circles until they are small. Reverse the shoulder rotations, circling your shoulders backward. Keep the rotations small and gradually increase their size until you reach maximum extension. After you complete your rotations, cross one arm over your chest parallel to the ground. Use the other arm to pull from underneath across the body, to increase the stretch. Last, reach with one arm above the head and fold it down at the elbow to touch the back of the neck. Use the other arm to exert slight pressure at the elbow tip to stretch the shoulder.

The Lower Back   From the passive-outlet stance (see page 56), place your hands on your lower back. Circle your hips to your left and then reverse direction to your right. The idea is to limber your lower back gently.

The Wrists   Rotate your wrists to the left clockwise and counterclockwise. Then bend the wrists up and down.

The Hamstrings   From your passive-outlet stance, bend forward from the hips, bringing your hands toward your toes or the floor. Keep your knees straight. Stand up and shake the legs out. Repeat the stretch, trying to extend farther. Next take a step forward with one leg, keeping that leg straight. Bend forward from the hips and reach your hands to the floor. Last, spread your legs in a partial split as far as you are comfortable. Be careful with this stretch not to lose control of the stretch and your balance, which can result in an injury. Bend forward and touch the ground if you can. Do not bounce.

The Groin   Sit with your legs in a butterfly position, the bottom edges of your feet together and your knees out to the sides. Gently push down on your inner thighs with your elbows or hands.

The Hips   From the groin-stretch position, take one leg back behind you so your front leg is bent approximately 90 degrees and your rear leg is now bent 90 degrees but behind you. Try to keep the rear leg's heel as close as possible to your buttocks. Gently bend forward to stretch the forward leg's hip flexors. Repeat with the other leg.

The Quadriceps   From the hip-stretch position, lean backward as far as you are comfortable to stretch the quadriceps. Some people are flexible enough to lean all the way back until touching their backs to the floor. Try to keep the rear leg's heel close to your buttock to alleviate pressure on the knee.

The Calves Stand up and assume your fighting stance. Place your feet parallel and facing forward. To stretch you rear calf, lean forward, placing your palms against a wall. Keep the back heel against the ground.

After completing your workout, cool down by stretching, using the same routine as above to enhance your flexibility and help rid your muscles of lactic acid, a buildup of toxic by-products of energy production.

Getting in Shape

Close-quarters combat is strenuous and grueling. Physical exhaustion combined with mental taxation from fear can immediately sap your ability and, more important, your will to fight. Optimally, you should augment your *krav maga* training plan with physical training that includes the following:

Aerobic Training Aerobic exercise, such as running, cycling, marching, or swimming, increases your cardiovascular efficiency and the ability of your body to transport and absorb oxygen. Aim for 20 to 40 minutes of effort 3 to 4 times a week. Jumping rope is also a great form of conditioning. Last, doing 20 minutes of concentrated *retzev* with good form will also give you a good aerobic workout.

Anaerobic Training Complete a strengthening session 3 to 4 times a week, using weights and your body weight as resistance. Perform each exercise until exhaustion, the point when you can't perform an additional repetition. Complete 8 to 15 reps of the following exercises: push-ups, crunches, dips, pull-ups, bench presses, military presses, and squats. To specifically enhance your fighting strength and stamina, I recommend a "high intensity" superset weight training program involving 2–3 sets of 8–15 reps. Each set requires you to tax your targeted muscle group to failure while paying strict attention to your form. You should use a heavy enough weight where you can do at least 8 reps but no more than 15 without struggling to complete the last rep within that range. Rather than resting between sets, reduce the weight by about 20 percent and immediately compete your second or third sets. The only rest is the time it takes to reduce the weight on the bar, machine, or dumbbells. In other words, if you are using 50 pounds for the first set, you should use 40 pounds for the second set, and 30 pounds for the third.

Mental Training   Visualize potential threatening encounters—and your reactions to them—as often as possible. Whenever you find yourself with free time, such as when you are sitting in your car during your commute to work, think of various situations ranging from purse snatchings to terrorist attacks. Imagine every detail—the sights, sounds, smells, and so on. Imagine how you respond to the threat, the techniques you use, and how the attacker responds to those techniques. Repeat similar scenarios until they become second-nature to you, and then invent new ones. The more often you think about how you will respond to a threat, the more instinctively you will respond in real life.

The *Kravist* Workouts

The *kravist* training plan includes 3 to 4 hours of concentrated training per week to help you hone your skills, tone your body, and build cardiovascular endurance. Each workout lasts roughly one to one and a half hours. You'll practice 3 to 4 days a week, with one rest day between workouts. If you visit a fitness facility, you can fit in the *krav maga* training before or after your regular fitness training. During the twelve-week plan, you will complete a number of drills, exercise, and workouts, both alone and with a partner.

Training Solo

Practicing techniques in the air develops muscle memory through repetitive movements. You must train alone to develop your *ret-zev* or continuous-motion combative movements. Practicing your movements in front of a mirror is one of the best methods to accomplish correct form and fluidity. Watching yourself will improve your movements and keep your head sighted on your opponent. The training plan includes the following workouts without a partner:

Balance exercises. Practice the following balance exercises before your *krav maga* training session to enhance your coordination and body control. When you first try these exercises, keep your hands out to your side for maximum balance. As your balance improves, position your hands in your outlet stance and try to avoid extending your arms. Extending your arms to your sides when kicking is a common mistake that telegraphs your movements to your opponent (always keep your arms *up* in your outlet stance!). Note that your center of gravity is just below your navel. If you begin to lose your balance, drop your center of gravity by bending your knees and widening your stance.

1. Balancing from your extended straight-knee position and then your roundhouse-knee position with one leg in the air.

2. Come into an airplane position with one leg extended, one leg raised behind, and your arms spread out to your sides.

3. Raise yourself on one leg and extend it forward, to the side, and then to the rear without letting your foot

touch the ground. These movements along with base leg pivots mimic your straight, side, and defense rear kicks.

4. Complete *retzev* movements using every technique you have learned for several minutes to practice your balance, combatives form, fluidity, and stamina.

Shadow boxing in front of a mirror. Practice your striking combinations from chapter 4 from both the left- and right-outlet stance using all types and combinations of punches and elbows in front of a mirror. In essence, you are your opponent in the mirror. Watch for good form and repeat a movement if you observe yourself incorrectly performing a technique. Be careful not to hyperextend your elbows.

Punch feints. Feints deceive your opponent of your true intention and force him to react using an improper defense as you follow through with the actual combative. They can be difficult to master, but devastating to your opponent if employed properly. The key is to sell the feint by using one fluid movement instead of two. Convince your opponent you are going to do one combative, but instead you do another. For example, pretend you are going to launch a roundhouse kick. Begin the movement as you normally would, but, mid-motion transform the kick into a straight kick.

Training Drills with a Partner

You'll need a training partner to move past the theory stage (practicing in the air) and put the movements into practice. As you work with a partner, you will develop trust, which will enhance your ability to work with each other. Training with multiple partners is also beneficial for the obvious reason that no two people move exactly alike. Variations will improve your reactions. In addition, someone with longer limbs will execute attacks and defenses differently than someone with shorter limbs. Men and women should train with each other interchangeably.

You should coordinate training with your partner to ensure maximum training benefit. Designate who will perform the specific defensive technique against the corresponding mock attack. After sufficient practice and familiarity with a given technique, series of techniques, and overall training concept, introduce variations. Training variations with a partner come in two training phases: (1) *limited*—in which you predetermine how your partner will attack and vary the attacks, and (2) *unlimited*—you know a variation will come but do not necessarily know how or when.

Limited training, for example, might include practicing defenses against preset punch attacks. For example, you know your partner is going to attack with a straight right punch to your head. In the next drill, your partner, either following the direction of an instructor or on his own initiative, informs you that he will throw a right roundhouse punch to your head. The point is that you *always know* what is coming.

Unlimited open training allows your training to encompass the entire scope of a technique or number of techniques. *Unlimited open training* is used at the most advanced levels to represent the street's unexpected dangers. Using our above example, the exercise changes for unlimited open-training punch attacks as follows: you do not know which arm will launch the attack (right or left), what type of attack (straight, roundhouse, uppercut, or modifications of these), or the attack angle (straight or from an "off angle"), and height (high or low). The point is that you *do not know* what is coming!

The training plans include the following partner drills.

Punch defense drills. These drills focus on specific punch defenses from chapter 4. For these movements, make sure you and your partner execute your respective part of the drill: one attacks and the other defends. After you become confident in the technique, begin to add additional *retzev* counterattacks using everything you have learned. Both of you should begin in left-outlet stances, except in the first two drills, where the opponents begin in passive-outlet stances (for practice purposes only).

Kick/knee defense drills. Your partner kicks as you defend against the kick. Partners should kick with control and accuracy to ensure safety and allow the drill to function properly. Shin guards are recommended. Over time you may wish to discard them and condition your legs to different levels of impact.

Kick/knee strikes and combination pad work. Practice your kicks and knees by connecting with a pad your partner holds. Be careful not to hyperextend your elbows and knees. To complete these drills, you will need focus mitts, handshields, or "muy thai"–type pads. (See the appendix for ordering information).

Work in coordination with your partner for effective pad work. (A heavy bag also serves as a good training tool.) Your partner determines your strike combinations by holding the pads in a certain manner. For example, if your partner holds his arms straight out with the front of the pads facing you, he is signaling for straight punches, palm heels, and forearm strikes. If your partner turns the pads inward so that his palms face each other, he is signaling for hook punches or horizontal elbows and chops. If the pads are held with the fronts facing the ground, they are positioned for uppercut punches and vertical elbows. If held low enough, the pads can be used for knee strikes. With practice, your partner will meet your strikes midmotion with the pad. For the pad work section of each workout, practice the suggested strikes for as long as it takes to break a good sweat. By the time you finish, you should be breathing heavily and your muscles should feel fatigued.

As you strike the pad, emphasize proper hip and shoulder movements. Drive your attack(s) directly through the target. Use proper footwork to move in and out; especially when leading with your forward arm for straight punches. Partners using strong, all-strike pad work should work in concert, and the pad holder may begin to move the hand pads and deliver counterattacks when the other partner leaves himself unprotected.

Use all of your strikes and combinations for pad-work drills. You may wish to use a large kicking shield for kicks, knees, and body attacks. The shield can also be raised to allow for straight punches. Muy thai–type striking pads are good for punches, elbows, knees, and medium and high roundhouse kicks. Consult the resource list in the appendix for ordering information.

Timing drills. Timing drills develop your self-defense capabilities and fighting prowess. For these drills you will spar slowly with your partner. As your partner delivers a punch or kick, you will move away, out of the kick's reach, and then follow up with your own punch or kick. Specific timing drills are described in the twelve-week plan. Refer to previous chapters for descriptions for each technique.

Your Twelve-week Program.

After a warmup, practice the following drills 3 to 4 times a week, with a day of rest between workouts. Combine the upper-body combative drills in column 1, lower-body combative drills in column 2, and the combination drills in column 3 into one comprehensive workout. As you'll see, some drills are performed solo, and others with a partner. Some are done with a training pad. Each week your *kravist* workout will become somewhat longer and more intense as you build your skills and fitness.

Schedule	Upper Body Combative Drills	Lower Body Combative Drills	Combinations
WEEK 1 Use proper footwork to move in and out with combinations. You may also close your eyes to perform combinations by envisioning boxing movements. For lateral movements (from the left-outlet stance), draw your right foot back to break the angle followed by the left foot. Obviously, do the opposite movements from a right-outlet stance.	SOLO *From the left-outlet stance:* • 15 repetitions of the straight front punch • 15 repetitions of the straight rear punch • 15 repetitions of the straight front/rear-punch combination with step and pivot. • Repeat each drill from the right-outlet stance WITH A PARTNER • 360-degree defense against outside strikes when one partner defends against outside attacks (with no counterstrike). Make sure the "attacking" partner executing the mock attack delivers wide deliberate outside strikes. (Note: the attacking partner does not use straight punches.)	SOLO *From the left-outlet stance*: • 15 repetitions of the straight front kick • 15 repetitions of the straight front knee • 15 repetitions of the straight rear kick • 15 repetitions of the straight rear knee • 15 repetitions of the straight rear/front-kick combination with proper pivoting, using the rear leg to initiate • 15 repetitions of the straight rear/front-knee combination with proper pivoting, using the rear leg to initiate WITH A PARTNER • Shin deflection to parry the opponent's kicking leg (straight kick defense #1) *Partner pad work:* Straight front and rear kick and straight kick with the rear leg	SOLO *From the left-outlet stance*: • 15 repetitions of the straight rear kick with a step forward (into opposite outlet stance) and punch with the same-side arm as the kick • 15 repetitions of the straight rear knee with a step forward (into opposite outlet stance) and punch with the same-side arm as the kick • Repeat each drill from the right-outlet stance 5 minutes of *retzev*, using punches, knees, and kicks in one continuous motion.

Schedule	Upper Body Combative Drills	Lower Body Combative Drills	Combinations
	Partner pad work: The straight front/rear-punch combination with step and pivot	and then knee with other leg	
WEEK 2	SOLO • Repeat week 1, using 5 repetitions for each punch and punch combination from both outlet stances *From the left-outlet stance:* • 15 repetitions of the front roundhouse punch • 15 repetitions of the front horizontal elbow • 15 repetitions of the rear roundhouse punch • 15 repetitions of the rear horizontal elbow • 10 repetitions of the front/rear-punch roundhouse combination, with proper pivoting. • 10 repetitions of the front/rear horizontal-elbow *(Cont'd)*	SOLO • Repeat week 1, using 10 repetitions for each kick from both outlet stances *From the left-outlet stance:* • 15 repetitions of the straight kick low/high combinations with the same leg front straight kick and rear (the leg should briefly touch the ground in between the respective kicks) WITH A PARTNER • Defend against the opponent's kicking leg (shin deflection) *Partner pad work:* Straight kick to groin from rear and knee to head with same leg	SOLO • Repeat week 1, using 10 repetitions for each punch/kick combination from both outlet stances. *From the left-outlet stance:* • 15 repetitions of the straight front kick with the front leg, using the forward leg shuffle (stepping the rear foot to where the front foot was as you slide forward) to step and deliver the straight front punch with same side • 15 repetitions of the straight front kick with the front leg, using the forward leg shuffle to step and deliver the straight front/rear-punch combination *(Cont'd)*

Schedule	Upper Body Combative Drills	Lower Body Combative Drills	Combinations
	combination, with proper pivoting • 15 repetitions of the lateral elbow to each side • Repeat each drill from the right-outlet stance WITH A PARTNER • 360-degree defense with simultaneous counterattack. This is a modification of the drill from week 1; however, one partner defends against outside strikes delivering simultaneous counterpunches or strikes. Be careful not to injure your partner performing the mock attack. The partner conducting the mock attack may wish to hold a pad or the nonattacking hand out for a target (obviously, not in front of the face)		• Repeat each drill from the right-outlet stance 6 minutes of *retzev*, using straight punches, elbows, knees, and kicks

Schedule	Upper Body Combative Drills	Lower Body Combative Drills	Combinations
	Partner pad work: The front/rear-roundhouse-punch combination high and low		
WEEK 3	SOLO Repeat weeks 1–2, using 5 repetitions for each punch and punch combination from both outlet stances *From the left-outlet stance:* • 15 repetitions of the front low roundhouse punch • 15 repetitions of the rear low roundhouse punch • 10 repetitions of the low front/rear round-house-punch combination with proper pivoting • Repeat each drill from the right-outlet stance. The front/rear-round-house-punch combination at the same level and then *(Cont'd)*	SOLO Repeat weeks 1–2, using 5 repetitions for each kick and kick combination from both outlet stances. *From the left-outlet stance:* • 15 repetitions of the sidekick, kicking with the front leg using *glicha* (the base leg slides) • Repeat each drill from the right-outlet stance WITH A PARTNER • Inside deflection against the high kick turning the forearm inside to misdirect the kick. Similar to the uppercut punch defense. *Partner pad work:* Side and rear defensive kicks	SOLO Repeat weeks 1–2, using 5 repetitions • 15 repetitions of the sidekick, kicking with the front leg using *glicha* (the base leg slides) followed by the reverse backfist • 6 minutes of *retzev*, using punches, elbows, knees, and kicks, followed by a same-side backfist and sidekick combination. Note: from the back fist, transition immediately into punches, knees, and kicks

Schedule	Upper Body Combative Drills	Lower Body Combative Drills	Combinations
	alternate high and low punches with opposite arms • The front/rear uppercut-punch combination WITH A PARTNER • Inside punch-deflection drill (using palm heel and minimal movement). One partner practices straight punches at half-speed while the other partner deflects. Be sure to deliver proper punches under maximum control to enable the drill while preventing injury • Blocks against low punches ("gunting" or Position 4 of 360-degree defense) when your partner delivers straight punches to the body *Partner pad work*: The front/rear uppercut combination		

Schedule	Upper Body Combative Drills	Lower Body Combative Drills	Combinations
WEEK 4	SOLO Repeat weeks 1–3, using 5 repetitions for each punch and punch combination from both outlet stances *From the left-outlet stance*: • 15 repetitions of the rear horizontal elbow. Repeat the drill over both your left and right shoulders • 10 repetitions combining left and right reverse horizontal elbows • Repeat each drill from the right-outlet stance **WITH A PARTNER** • Lateral-movement body defenses (no contact is made) to the dead and live sides of the your attacking partner, who throws a straight punch with either arm. The punching arm your attacker uses will *(Cont'd)*	SOLO Repeat weeks 1–3, using 5 repetitions for each kick and kick combination from both outlet stances • 15 repetitions with the side kick, kicking with the front leg, using *secoul* (a step through with the front leg and then the base leg to give the kick greater distance) • 15 repetitions of the rear defensive kick • Repeat each drill from the right-outlet stance **WITH A PARTNER** • Body defense with hand deflection with hand deflection (inside knee/shin bar) *Partner Pad work*: Front and rear roundhouse kicks	SOLO Repeat weeks 1–3, using 5 repetitions for each punch and kick combination from both outlet stances • 15 repetitions of the sidekick, kicking with the front leg using *glicha* (the base leg slides) followed by the reverse hammerfist. • 7 minutes of *retzev*, using punches, elbows, knees, and kicks in all directions (specifically including the side-kick/back-fist combination) Note: from the back fist, transition immediately into punches, knees, and kicks

Schedule	Upper Body Combative Drills	Lower Body Combative Drills	Combinations
	determine his dead and live side. The defender should use left/right body defensive punches and hook punches to the body *Partner pad work*: Low straight punches with body defense		
WEEK 5	SOLO Repeat weeks 1–4, using 4 repetitions for each punch and punch combination from both outlet stances *From the left outlet stance*: • 15 repetitions of the front uppercut punch • 15 repetitions of the front uppercut elbow • 15 repetitions of the rear uppercut punch • 15 repetitions of the rear uppercut elbow • 10 repetitions of the front/ rear uppercut combination with proper pivoting • Repeat each	SOLO Repeat weeks 1–4, using 4 repetitions for each kick and kick combination from both outlet stances *From the left-outlet stance*: • 15 repetitions of the front roundhouse kick, using proper pivot step with the base (rear) leg • 15 repetitions of the front roundhouse knee, using proper pivot with the base (rear) leg • 15 repetitions of the rear roundhouse kick, using proper pivot step with the base (front) leg	SOLO Repeat weeks 1–4, using 4 repetitions for each kick and kick combination from both outlet stances *From the left-outlet stance*: • 15 repetitions of the straight kick with the front leg, using the forward leg shuffle to step and punch with same-side arm, followed by a rear straight punch, a forward horizontal elbow, a rear horizontal elbow, and a rear knee • Repeat the drill from the left- outlet stance • 8 minutes of *retzev*, using

Schedule	Upper Body Combative Drills	Lower Body Combative Drills	Combinations
	drill from the right-outlet stance	• 15 repetitions of the rear roundhouse knee, using proper pivot step with the base (front) leg	punches, elbows, knees, and kicks in all directions
	WITH A PARTNER • Upper body retreating defenses using a backward lean against straight and roundhouse punches without stepping back. One partner uses upper-body defense movements to avoid the combatives thrown by the other partner. Exert maximum control and perform the drill at a manageable speed	• 10 repetitions of the front/rear roundhouse-kick combination with proper pivoting • 10 repetitions of the front/rear roundhouse knee combination with proper pivoting • Repeat each drill from the right-outlet stance	**WITH A PARTNER** • Partners use timing to exchange kicks (three varieties— straight, side, and roundhouse) without contact for five minutes. One partner follows through with a kick while the other partner retreats using a body defense and then delivers his own kick. In short, partners trade kicks *with no contact*. As one partner is withdrawing his kick, the other partner initiates his. Precision, control, and timing are the focus
	Partner pad work: Low roundhouse punch and then high roundhouse with same arm	**WITH A PARTNER** • Defenses against knees: the partner who is defending closes distance with a cross brace (inside knee/shin bar) with body weight pressing against the attacker's knee, with simultaneous upper-body combatives	
		Partner pad work: Combination kicks using straight, round-house, side, and rear defensive kicks	

Schedule	Upper Body Combative Drills	Lower Body Combative Drills	Combinations
Week 6	Solo Repeat weeks 1–5, using 3 repetitions for each punch and punch combination from both outlet stances *From the left-outlet stance*: • 15 repetitions of the straight punch and roundhouse punch or horizontal elbow combination with the same arm • 10 repetitions of the straight punch and roundhouse punch or horizontal elbow followed by a rear roundhouse punch or horizontal elbow • Repeat each drill from the right-outlet stance *Partner pad work*: Straight punch and horizontal elbow combination with the same arm	Solo Repeat week 1–5, using 3 repetitions for each kick and kick combination from both outlet stances *From the left-outlet stance*: • 10 repetitions of the straight kick with the rear leg while stepping forward into rear round-house kick with the opposite (rear) leg; • 10 repetitions of the straight knee with the rear leg while stepping forward into rear knee kick the opposite (rear) leg; • Repeat each drill from the right-outlet stance With a Partner • Defense against knees: the partner who is defending gunts with the elbows against the other partner's thighs. Use caution. Once comfortable with the drill, add *retzev* combatives	Solo Repeat week 1–5, using 3 repetitions for each punch and kick combination from both outlet stances With a Partner • Partners use timing to exchange kicks (three varieties—straight, side, and roundhouse) without contact for five minutes. One partner follows through with a kick while the other partner retreats, using a body defense and then delivers his own kick. In short, partners trade kicks *with no contact*. As one partner is withdrawing his kick, the other partner initiates his. Precision, control, and timing are the focus • 15 repetitions of the round-house kick with the front leg, followed by a straight front-arm punch, followed by a

Schedule	Upper Body Combative Drills	Lower Body Combative Drills	Combinations
			straight rear-arm punch, followed by a rear round-house kick • Repeat each drill from the right-outlet stance • 9 minutes of *retzev*, using punches, elbows, knees, and kicks in all directions *Partner pad work:* One partner holds a shield and feigns a punching motion. The other partner kicks the shield with control. This is not a power-centric drill. Remember, the partner holding the shield is extending himself to punch, making the body vulnerable behind the shield. This drill simulates a timing kick to preempt an incoming straight or hook punch One partner holds a hand pad (away from the face) and simulates a hook *(Cont'd)*

Schedule	Upper Body Combative Drills	Lower Body Combative Drills	Combinations
			punch. The defending partner uses timing to deliver a straight punch to the pad. This drill simulates a simultaneous defense and attack to prevent a circular or looping type of attack
WEEK 7	SOLO Repeat weeks 1–6, using 3 repetitions for each punch and punch combination from both outlet stances. *From the left-outlet stance:* • 15 repetitions of the front straight punch followed by front roundhouse punch with forward arm and uppercut with rear arm • 15 repetitions of the over-the-top elbow with the front arm • 15 repetitions of the over-the-top elbow with the rear arm • 10 repetitions of the over-the-top front and	SOLO Repeat week 1–6 using 3 repetitions for each kick and kick combination from both outlet stances. *From the left-outlet stance:* • 15 repetitions of the front/rear roundhouse combination • Repeat the drill from the right-outlet stance WITH A PARTNER • Defense against knees—partner defending gunts with the elbows against the attacker partner's thighs. Use caution. Note: once comfortable, add *retzev* combatives. Straight kick	SOLO Repeat week 1–6 using 3 repetitions for each kick and kick combination from both outlet stances. Try combining all these drills together, adding two additional combatives, then four additional combatives, then six additional combatives, and so on to build your *retzev*. Any combination of these movements and others you have (combining different techniques will also test how well you have learned the fundamentals) • 10 minutes of *retzev*, using punches, elbows,

Schedule	Upper Body Combative Drills	Lower Body Combative Drills	Combinations
	rear elbow combination • Repeat each drill from the right-outlet stance WITH A PARTNER • Double parry against straight punches with simultaneous straight kick or knee. One partner delivers a front/rear straight combination while the other partner defends using an inside block to parry. The defending partner throws a simultaneous straight knee or kick without making contact *Partner pad work:* Straight punch and horizontal roundhouse combination with the same arm	with the front leg using shuffle into rear round-house kick with the rear leg WITH A PARTNER • *Defenses Against the Side Kick—* Stop kick against the opponent's kicking leg or Side Kick Defense against side kick	knees, and kicks in all directions
WEEK 8	SOLO Repeat weeks 1–7, using 3 repetitions for each punch and punch combination *(Cont'd)*	SOLO Repeat weeks 1–7, using 3 repetitions for each kick and kick combination from both outlet stances. *(Cont'd)*	SOLO Repeat weeks 1–7, using 3 repetitions for each kick and kick combination from both outlet stances. Combine *(Cont'd)*

Schedule	Upper Body Combative Drills	Lower Body Combative Drills	Combinations
	from both outlet stances. *From the left-outlet stance:* • 15 repetitions of the front straight punch, followed by a front uppercut punch, followed by a roundhouse punch with rear arm • Repeat from the right-outlet stance **WITH A PARTNER** • A variation of the week 7 drill using a two-handed sliding block with knee attack (use the front knee for speed with *glicha* or the rear knee for power) • Move to the dead side against a left punch with the front knee (attacker and defender are both in the left side forward-outlet stance) • Move to the live side against a right punch with the rear knee (attacker and defender both are in the left side forward-outlet stance)	*From the left-outlet stance:* • 15 repetitions of the high/low roundhouse combination with same leg and low/high roundhouse combination with same leg • Repeat each drill from the right-outlet stance	all these drills together, adding two additional combatives, then four additional combatives, then six additional combatives, and so on. Any combination of these movements and others you have learned (combining different techniques will also test how well you have learned the fundamentals.) • 11 minutes of *retzev*, using punches, elbows, knees, and kicks in all directions

Schedule	Upper Body Combative Drills	Lower Body Combative Drills	Combinations
	Partner pad work: Roundhouse punch with forward arm and straight punch with the rear arm		
WEEK 9	SOLO Repeat weeks 1–8, using 2 repetitions for each punch and punch combination from both outlet stances. *From the left-outlet stance:* • Any combination of all the previous upper-body combatives without pause (helping to establish a *retzev* base) • Repeat from the right-outlet stance WITH A PARTNER • Inside same-side sliding defense against a straight punch (defender keeps elbow down and parries/ slides over the top of the punch to *(Cont'd)*	SOLO Repeat weeks 1–8, using 2 repetitions for each kick and kick combination from both outlet stance. *From the left-outlet stance:* • 15 repetitions of the intercepting side kick against the opponent's straight kicking leg • Repeat the drill from the right-outlet stance	SOLO 12 minutes of *retzev*, using punches, elbows, knees, and kicks in all directions Repeat weeks 1–8, using 2 repetitions for each kick and kick combination from both outlet stances WITH A PARTNER • From the left-outlet stance, the defender traps the attacker's arms (also standing in an outlet stance) inward and executes offensive knee with proper pivot, pulling attacker's arms to generate additional momentum *Defenses Against Combinations:* • Mentally visualize the *(Cont'd)*

Schedule	Upper Body Combative Drills	Lower Body Combative Drills	Combinations
	deliver inverted punch) *Partner pad work*: Round house punch with forward arm and uppercut with rear arm		defenses you would use against all of the combinations you have learned. Two examples include: • Defend against a straight kick to the groin and punch to the face (inside deflections and counterattacks) • Defend against a roundhouse kick at varying heights and punches that may be used in combination following the kick
WEEK 10	SOLO Repeat weeks 1–8, using 2 repetitions for each punch and punch combination from both outlet stances. *From the left-outlet stance*: • Feinting roundhouse punch into straight punch • Repeat the drill from the right-outlet stance	SOLO Repeat weeks 1–8, using 2 repetitions for each kick and kick combination from both outlet stances. *From the left-outlet stance*: • Roundhouse kick feint into straight kick using the rear leg • Repeat the drill from the right-outlet stance	SOLO Repeat weeks 1–8, using 2 repetitions for each kick and kick combination from both outlet stances • 13 minutes of *retzev*, using punches, elbows, knees, and kicks in all directions WITH A PARTNER • From the outlet stance, the defender splits the attacker's arms (also standing in an

Schedule	Upper Body Combative Drills	Lower Body Combative Drills	Combinations
	WITH A PARTNER Inside punch defense against a right punch (from partner's left-outlet stance) pinning the arm at the crook and continuing with a straight punch with the opposite arm and other combatives. The same basic defense is available with slight modification if the attacker is in the right-outlet stance and punches with his right. *Partner pad work*: Straight punch with forward arm and uppercut with same arm	**WITH A PARTNER** *Defenses against the side kick.* Shin deflection variation (straight kick defense) Note: Once comfortable, add *retzev* combatives	outlet stance), using a wedge motion by placing the palms together and diving inward while executing the offensive rear knee *Body absorption drill:* Partner works at moving with strikes and absorbing blows while exhaling. The drill can also be performed with the eyes closed (partners must take careful control of strikes)
WEEK 11	**SOLO** • Repeat weeks 1–8, ... 2 repetitions • 15 repetitions of feinting the straight punch in roundhouse punch; **WITH A PARTNER** Partness stand side to side facing in opposite directions • Defense against outside straight *(Cont'd)*	**SOLO** • Repeat weeks 1–8, ... 2 repetitions • 15 repetitions of feinting the roundhouse kick into straight kick using either leg **WITH A PARTNER** • *Defenses against the low roundhouse kick* using the forward leg deflection both opening-up and closing inside	**SOLO** • Repeat weeks 1–8, ... 2 repetitions • 14 minutes of *retzev,* using punches, elbows, knees, and kicks in all directions **WITH A PARTNER** • *Defenses against a surprise attack:* • Under strict control, partners practice surprise attacks from all *(Cont'd)*

Schedule	Upper Body Combative Drills	Lower Body Combative Drills	Combinations
	punches, using similar 360-degree deflection defense (usually block with position 3) and employing immediate counterstrikes including: • Low round-house punch or chop to the opponent's kidneys (by stepping through with the far leg), followed by additional combatives • Roundhouse knee to kidneys with additional combatives *Partner pad work*: Roundhouse punch with forward arm and uppercut with rear arm		angles, including strikes and grabs. One partner uses a deliberate slow attack while the other partner defends, optimally using a specific corresponding defense followed by a *retzev* counterattack, using no fewer than five counterstrikes
WEEK 12	SOLO • Feinting straight punch into uppercut; WITH A PARTNER • A timing or preemptive kick defense using the front leg against a straight or hook punch (opponent uses either arm) kicking the	SOLO • Straight kick feint into side kick using the rear leg WITH A PARTNER • *Defenses against the roundhouse kick by* stepping out and to the side away from the kick to catch the opponent's leg;	SOLO • Repeat weeks 1–8, using 2 repetitions for each kick and kick combination from both outlet stances. • 15 minutes of *retzev*, using punches, elbows, knees, and kicks in all directions

Schedule	Upper Body Combative Drills	Lower Body Combative Drills	Combinations
	opponent's groin or midsection. The defender uses the kick's superior reach to stop the attacker, followed by additional combatives. If the defender is to the side, use the side kick. This is a timing drill. Be sure to exert maximum control making no contact • From the left-outlet stance, the defender traps the attacker's arms (also standing in an outlet stance) inward and executes offensive knee with proper pivot, pulling attacker's arms to generate additional momentum *Partner pad work*: • Uppercut with forward arm and roundhouse with same arm • Uppercut with forward arm and roundhouse with rear arm • Upper cut into straight punch. • Combinations of the previous 11 weeks	• *Defenses against the roundhouse kick* by blocking with the forearms using the proper angle and counterstrikes against high kicks. • Straight kick into roundhouse using the front leg • Roundhouse kick into straight punch (kick does not land).	WITH A PARTNER • *Defenses against retzev ("continuous motion") attacks* • This drill uses the defenses that you know to defend your partner's continuous motion attacks. This is a highly beneficial drill for both partners. • This drill will quickly assert the importance of *retzev's* dominance in a fight. Moreover, you will appreciate the role of simultaneous (or near simultaneous) defense and attack. The defender can stand against the wall to prevent the tendency to retreat

Twelve Weeks and Beyond

Once you have completed the twelve-week program, continue to practice *krav maga*, using the drills from the program as a practice guide. Combine those drills with the following sample workouts and drills, which will help you to take your *krav maga* training to the next level.

Total Body Workout

This sample workout combines all the combatives you have learned and forces you to recall what combatives are now in your arsenal.

1. Jumping rope for three minutes. Stay on the balls of your feet, not your heels. As you grow more proficient. include different steps and crisscrossing the rope.
2. Gentle stretching for fifteen minutes.
3. Up-downs (dropping your body to the ground similar to a forward soft-fall break and exploding to your feet immediately only to drop again) for three minutes.
4. Shadow or *tzel* box for three minutes. Incorporate continuous strikes and body defenses. Be sure to use proper form, especially your pivots, and follow-through with each punch but do not lock your elbows.
5. Twenty push-ups.
6. Shadow infighting with elbows and knees for three minutes. This is the same drill as shadow boxing except you use your elbows and knees.
7. Twenty sit-ups.
8. Kicks for three minutes using proper pivots and weight shifts. Be careful not to lock your legs.
9. *Reztev* with all body strikes for three minutes slowly.
10. *Retvez* with all body strikes for three minutes quickly.

Play Fighting with a Partner

Play fighting (*mista krav* or "controlled light") develops your fighting technique through *retzev*. Play fighting will improve your coordination, stamina, and overall fighting prowess. You'll spar with your partner, using the techniques you know and countering the techniques your partner throws at you. Play fighting is not full-contact power sparring but instead focuses on deliberate, slow movements. You can increase the speed as your skill set improves, but keep power to a minimum.

The following "play-fighting" drills will put into action all the combatives and corresponding defenses you have learned.

1. Both partners stand close and attempt to take one another off balance.
2. Each partner tries to slap the other partner's knees using defenses and attacks.
3. Slow infighting with elbows and knees.
4. Practice a timing technique with one partner using the superior reach of the legs against the other partner who is only using the upper body.
5. Practice the same legs-against-hands drill with one partner against the wall.
6. Practice a hands-against-hands drill, using timing, upper-body parry and body defenses, and boxing drills.
7. Practice a legs-against-legs drill, using timing and lower-body parry defenses.
8. Practice a knees-against-knees drill, using timing and lower-body parry defenses.
9. Practice groundwork. Similar to play fighting while standing, you'll call upon your *krav maga* techniques as you lie on the ground. In particular, you do not want an attacker to grab hold and control any of your limbs. The same combative techniques will apply to ground situations, with minor modifications.

10. Practice play fighting using the hands and feet.

11. Practice with hands, legs, knees.

12. Practice with hands, legs, knees, and groundwork.

13. Practice with short punches, kicks, knees, elbows, head butts, catches, clinches, throws, and groundwork.

14. Practice defending against close punches, kicks, knees, elbows, clinches, throws, head butts, and groundwork, with counterattacks.

15. Practice with one partner using legs and hands against another partner who can only use hands.

16. Practice with one partner using legs and hands, but the other can only use legs.

17. One partner only attacks and the other partner only defends.

18. Attacker continues attack with defender reacting, and defender counters with a touch to the forehead or kick to the body, signaling for the attacker to retreat.

19. Play fight with the left or right hand only.

20. Touch boxing with gloves.

21. Utilize the longest (kicks) and intermediate (punches) strikes first and than close in for an infight with short-distance weapons (elbows and knees).

22. Defend against long- and intermediate-range attack and continue with counterattacks while closing the distance and continuing as an infight.

23. Practice falling to the ground in an advantageous position to make strong counterattacks against opponent's groin and legs.

24. Practice retreating with a straight punch and kick.

25. Clinch or trap opponent to neutralize or limit his ability to strike while delivering counterattacks.

Choke-Release and Bear-Hug-Release Drills Defender works with his partner to defend against chokes and grabs from different angles. The defender executes releases from all directions against chokes and bear hugs with control. A variation of the drill is to have the defender close his/her eyes.

The following two drills are designed for five people—one defender and four attackers. This configuration can simulate a group attack. As with all training drills, be careful to use slow and controlled movements and never use more than minimal power.

Four Against One Defending Controlled Attacks

Defender stands in the middle of four attackers in a diamond formation. One attacker is to the front, one to each side, and one to the rear. Attackers must coordinate the slow-speed, deliberate attacks. The defender executes blocks and counterattacks from all directions with control.

Choke and Bearhug Defense Drill from All Directions   Defender stands in the middle of four attackers in a diamond formation. The attackers must coordinate the attacks. The attackers choke and bearhug from different angles, and the defender executes releases from all directions against chokes and bear hugs with control. An advanced variation of the drill is to have the defender close his/her eyes.

A True *Kravist*

Now you know everything you need to know to begin your journey as a *kravist*, a true fighter. After completing the 12-week program, you should already be noticing some changes in your body, mind, and spirit. Perhaps you are already feeling more confident and more aware of your surroundings and possible dangerous situations. You should also see some positive changes in your body: more strength and firmness in your arms, legs, chest, back, and abdomen. Your balance and coordination have probably improved as well.

If you haven't done so already, sign up for some classes with a certified instructor. This will help you to fine-tune what you've learned from this book. A *krav maga* class will also provide you with plenty of sparring partners and a new community of like-minded people. I hope you become as close to your fellow *krav maga* students and instructors as I have come to mine, and that *krav maga* becomes not only a system of self-defense for you, but also a tight-knit circle of friends and companions.

So my friend, make this the beginning of a long, successful and safe journey. Continue always to improve your body and mind through *krav maga*. Remember to always use your fighting skills with great care, using the least amount of force necessary. I hope, of course, that you never have to use your skills, and that your life and the lives of your loved ones will never be threatened. I hope, too, that you will continue to enjoy the many challenges and rewards of living as a true *kravist*.

APPENDIX

Resources

To order protective padding and other supplies:

Asian World of Martial Arts
11601 Caroline Road
Philadelphia, PA 19154-2177
1-800-345-2962
www.amwa.com

Revgear Sports Co.
4406 Vanowen St.
Burbank, California 91505
1-800-767-8288
fax 1-818-847-1114
info@revgear.com
www.revgear.com

Israel Army Surplus
www.israelmilitary.com

To read more about krav maga and its history:

Fighting Fit: The Israel Defense Forces Guide to Physical Fitness and Self-Defense, by David Ben-Asher (Perigree, 1983)

The Making of Israel's Army, by Yigal Allon (Sphere Books Ltd., 1971)

The Israel Defense Forces Homepage: *www.idf.il*

The Israel Special Forces Homepage: *www.isayeret.com*

The International Defense Force Homepage: *www.i-d-f.com*

*To find a certified IKMA instructor
in the United States or abroad
and for more information:*

Israeli Krav Maga Association,
United States
www.israelikrav.com
PO Box 1234
Princeton, New Jersey 08540

The Israeli Krav Maga Association
www.kravmagaisraeli.com
PO Box 1103
Netanya
Israel

*For defensive tactics and protective
services:*
Hammerhead, LLC
100 Overlook Center, Suite 102
Princeton, New Jersey 08540
www.hammerheadops.com

ABOUT THE AUTHOR

David Kahn is one of America's leading experts in *krav maga*. After years of intensive training in Israel under Grandmaster Haim Gidon of the Israeli Krav Maga Association (IKMA) and having received his IKMA advanced blackbelt teaching certification, David now sits on the Association's board of directors as its only American representative.

David has been featured in *USA Today*, the *New Yorker*, and elsewhere, and was recently named a "Top Workout Guru" in *New York* magazine. He is founder and director of the *krav maga* program at the 92nd Street Y and also teaches at David Barton Gyms and elsewhere. His trainees include federal, state, and local law-enforcement professionals, as well as executives, celebrities, fitness enthusiasts, senior citizens, and others. A graduate of Princeton University, David is a cofounder of *HAMMERHEAD* Security Consulting. He lives in New Jersey.